T0259347

Innovations in the Cavus Foot Deformity

Editor

ANISH RAJ KADAKIA

FOOT AND ANKLE CLINICS

www.foot.theclinics.com

Consulting Editor
MARK S. MYERSON

December 2013 • Volume 18 • Number 4

ELSEVIER

1600 John F. Kennedy Boulevard • Suite 1800 • Philadelphia, Pennsylvania, 19103-2899

http://www.theclinics.com

FOOT AND ANKLE CLINICS Volume 18, Number 4
December 2013 ISSN 1083-7515, ISBN-13: 978-0-323-26096-1

Editor: Jennifer Flynn-Briggs

Foot and Ankle Clinics (ISSN 1083-7515) is published quarterly by Elsevier, Inc., 360 Park Avenue South, New York, NY 10010-1710. Months of issue are March, June, September, and December. Periodicals postage paid at New York, NY, and additional mailing offices. Subscription price per year is $315.00 (US individuals), $421.00 (US institutions), $155.00 (US students), $360.00 (Canadian individuals), $506.00 (Canadian institutions), $215.00 (Canadian students), $460.00 (foreign individuals), $506.00 (foreign institutions), and $215.00 (foreign students). To receive student/resident rate, orders must be accompanied by name of affiliated institution, date of term, and the *signature* of program/residency coordinator on institution letterhead. Orders will be billed at individual rate until proof of status is received. Foreign air speed delivery is included in all *Clinics* subscription prices. All prices are subject to change without notice. **POSTMASTER:** Send address changes to *Foot and Ankle Clinics*, Elsevier Health Sciences Division, Subscription Customer Service, 3251 Riverport Lane, Maryland Heights, MO 63043. **Customer Service: 1-800-654-2452 (US and Canada). From outside of the United States and Canada, call 314-447-8871. Fax: 314-447-8029. E-mail: JournalsCustomerService-usa@ elsevier.com (for print support); JournalsOnlineSupport-usa@elsevier.com (for online support).**

Reprints. For copies of 100 or more, of articles in this publication, please contact the Commercial Reprints Department, Elsevier Inc., 360 Park Avenue South, New York, NY 10010-1710. Tel.: 212-633-3874; Fax: 212-633-3820; E-mail: reprints@elsevier.com.

Printed and bound by CPI Group (UK) Ltd, Croydon, CR0 4YY

Transferred to digital print 2012

Contributors

CONSULTING EDITOR

MARK S. MYERSON, MD
Director, The Institute for Foot and Ankle Reconstruction, Mercy Medical Center, Baltimore, Maryland

EDITOR

ANISH RAJ KADAKIA, MD
Editor in Chief, Journal of Orthopedic Surgery and Research, Assistant Professor of Orthopedic Surgery, Northwestern University-Feinberg School of Medicine, Northwestern Memorial Hospital, Chicago, Illinois

AUTHORS

ALI ABBASIAN, FRCS (TR & ORTH)
Orthopaedic Foot and Ankle Surgeon, Guy's and St Thomas' Hospitals NHS Foundation Trust, London, United Kingdom

JASON T. BARITEAU, MD
Trauma Fellow, Department of Orthopaedic Surgery, The Warren Alpert Medical School, Brown University, Providence, Rhode Island

TRISTAN BARTON, MBChB, FRCS
Department of Trauma and Orthopaedics, Royal United Hospital Bath NHS Trust, Bath, United Kingdom

BRAD D. BLANKENHORN, MD, MS
Assistant Professor, Department of Orthopaedics and Rehabilitation, University of New Mexico School of Medicine, UNM Hospitals, Albuquerque, New Mexico

HILARY A. BOSMAN, BSc, MBBS, MRCS (Eng), FRCS (Tr & Orth)
Fellow in Foot and Ankle Surgery, Department of Trauma and Orthopaedics, Cambridge University Hospitals NHS Trust, Cambridge, United Kingdom

JAE-HO CHO, MD
Assistant Professor, Seoul Foot and Ankle Center, Inje University Seoul Paik Hospital, Seoul, Republic of Korea

MARTIN S. DICINTIO, CMT
Assistant Research Coordinator, Department of Pediatric Orthopaedic Surgery, Children's Hospital Medical Center of Akron, Akron, Ohio

CHRISTOPHER W. DIGIOVANNI, MD
Program Director and Chief, Foot and Ankle Service, Professor, Department of Orthopaedic Surgery, Rhode Island Hospital, The Warren Alpert Medical School, Brown

University; Department of Orthopaedic Surgery, University Orthopedics, Inc, Providence, Rhode Island

ABHIJIT GUHA, MBChB, FRCS(Orth)
University Hospital of Wales and Spire Cardiff Hospital, Llanishen, Cardiff, United Kingdom

ROBERT N. HENSINGER, MD
Department of Orthopaedic Surgery, The University of Michigan, Ann Arbor, Michigan

MARTIN HUBER, MD
Department for Foot and Ankle Surgery, Schulthess Klinik, Zürich, Switzerland

DAVID JONAH, MA
Medical Illustrator, Researcher, Belcamp, Maryland

KERWYN JONES, MD
Chairman, Department of Pediatric Orthopaedic Surgery, Children's Hospital Medical Center of Akron, Akron, Ohio

HONG-GEUN JUNG, MD, PhD
Department of Orthopedic Surgery, Konkuk University School of Medicine, Seoul, South Korea

BRANDON W. KING, MD
Department of Orthopaedic Surgery, The University of Michigan, Ann Arbor, Michigan

KANG LEE, MD
Assistant Professor, Department of Orthopaedic Surgery, Kangwon National University Hospital, Kangwon National University, Chuncheon, Republic of Korea

SANG-HUN LEE, MD
Department of Orthopedic Surgery, Konkuk University School of Medicine, Seoul, South Korea

WOO-CHUN LEE, MD, PhD
Professor, Seoul Foot and Ankle Center, Inje University Seoul Paik Hospital, Seoul, Republic of Korea

MARK S. MYERSON, MD
Director, The Institute for Foot and Ankle Reconstruction, Mercy Medical Center, Baltimore, Maryland

JONG-TAE PARK, MD
Department of Orthopedic Surgery, Good Samsun Hospital, Busan, South Korea

ANTHONY PERERA, MBChB, FRCS(Orth)
University Hospital of Wales and Spire Cardiff Hospital, Llanishen, Cardiff, United Kingdom

GREGORY POMEROY, MD
Director, New England Foot and Ankle Specialists, Department of Mercy Hospital, Clinical Associate Professor of Surgery, University of New England, Portland, Maine

ANDREW H.N. ROBINSON, BSc, MBBS, FRCS, FRCS (Orth)
Consultant Orthopaedic Foot and Ankle Surgeon, Department of Trauma and Orthopaedics, Cambridge University Hospitals NHS Trust, Cambridge, United Kingdom

JOSEF N. TOFTE, BA
Medical Student, Department of Orthopaedic Surgery, The Warren Alpert Medical School, Brown University, Providence, Rhode Island

KELLY L. VANDERHAVE, MD
Department of Orthopaedic Surgery, Carolinas Medical Center, Charlotte, North Carolina

DENNIS S. WEINER, MD
Chairman Emeritus, Department of Pediatric Orthopaedic Surgery, Children's Hospital Medical Center of Akron, Akron, Ohio

IAN WINSON, MBChB, FRCS
Department of Trauma and Orthopaedics, Avon Orthopaedic Centre, Southmead Hospital, Bristol, United Kingdom

JACOB R. ZIDE, MD
The Institute for Foot and Ankle Reconstruction, Mercy Medical Center, Baltimore, Maryland

Contents

The key to successful management of the cavovarus foot is identifying the pathoanatomy and dysfunction that are driving the deformity and producing the symptoms. There is no substitute for a thorough clinical evaluation of the foot, evaluating the static alignment and dynamic function. Plain films alone are not sufficient to determine the diagnosis, but they are necessary for procedure selection and correction planning. This is especially true for assessing the degree of hindfoot varus. Some issues are difficult to diagnose, and imaging plays an important role.

Idiopathic cavus deformity even in its mild form can result in several associated symptoms. Management of these symptoms without addressing the underlying biomechanical abnormality may result in failure of treatment. A careful clinical assessment is paramount.

This article reviews the role of cavus in foot and ankle injury and summarizes the current surgical and nonsurgical treatments. Recognition of foot position is crucial in the management of ankle instability associated with cavovarus. Correcting foot alignment with orthoses or surgery improves the mechanics of the ankle, reducing the risk of instability and potentially delaying the onset of posttraumatic ankle arthritis. Progressive steps in the correction alignment are described, with technical tips and strategies for dealing with chronic instability.

Adult cavovarus deformity patients present with rigid cavovarus deformity, where the correction can no longer be obtained using soft tissue procedures alone, and corrective arthrodesis or osteotomy must be performed to realign the deformity. Reconstructive surgeries for cavovarus foot deformities are variable and include hindfoot or midfoot osteotomy or arthrodesis, soft tissue release or lengthening, and tendon transfers. Recently

deformity. These patients are monitored long term because further treatment may be required.

This article reviews historical approaches to the various osteotomies in the treatment of rigid cavus feet in children, with an emphasis on the biplanar nature of historical osteotomies. The Akron dome midfoot osteotomy is performed at the apex of the rigid cavus deformity and allows for maximum correction in any plane, and for varus, valgus, dorsal, plantar, and rotational correction. In that regard, the Akron dome midfoot osteotomy provides the greatest amount of multiplanar correction. It does not, however, provide correction of hindfoot deformities or deformity distal to the neck of the metatarsal.

Cavovarus is a deformity commonly associated with a variety of underlying disorders, and treatment of severe cavovarus foot with an underlying progressive disorder is very challenging. Often patients have undergone some prior surgery at least once, with increased potential risk of neurovascular injury and breakdown of soft tissue. In addition, concomitant problems such as torsional malalignment and leg-length discrepancy should also be addressed to prevent recurrence and treatment failure. In this article, indications and an algorithmic approach with various osteotomies for the treatment of cavovarus deformity using external fixation are discussed in detail.

When the cavus foot has become rigid, midfoot and triple arthrodesis may be the only reasonable surgical options left. The apex of the deformity is multiplanar and some deformities may have more than one apex. The best outcomes are achieved with minimal shortening of the foot, so correction should be by rotation and translation and with minimal wedge resection wherever possible. Posterior tibial tendon transfer and peroneus longus transfer are nearly always required for correction. If the principles of soft tissue balancing are followed, arthrodesis is an excellent procedure despite the literature that states to the contrary.

FOOT AND ANKLE CLINICS

Erratum

An error was made in the September 2013 issue of Foot and Ankle Clinics (Volume 18, number 3) in the Contributors List, Table of Contents, and on pages 481–502. One of the author names for "Joint-preserving surgery of valgus ankle osteoarthritis" was listed incorrectly. The correct author name is Monika Horisberger.

Foot Ankle Clin N Am 18 (2013) xi
http://dx.doi.org/10.1016/j.fcl.2013.10.001
1083-7515/13/$ – see front matter © 2013 Elsevier Inc. All rights reserved.

foot.theclinics.com

Preface
The Cavus Foot

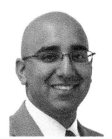

Anish Raj Kadakia, MD
Editor

Management of the cavovarus foot is challenging in determining which surgical procedures are required in addition to the complexity of the execution of the surgery itself. Surgical correction not only must address the bony abnormalities that are present but also requires attention to ligamentous stabilization and tendon rebalancing as well. In the setting of a severe deformity, surgical decision-making is facilitated; however, the decision to correct subtle deformity can be very challenging. We have formulated the articles to address the many controversial aspects in treating cavus foot deformity. The overall goal of the issue is not to delineate which procedures will provide the "perfect" x-ray. Our goal was to provide a thorough review of the pathology and surgical options to provide optimal function for the patient.

The authors in this issue of *Foot and Ankle Clinics of North America* are experts in dealing with cavovarus foot deformities. By sharing the knowledge and experience of our colleagues, each of us can expand our ability to understand and treat this condition. I would like to commend the authors on the tremendous time and effort that they put forth in preparation of their articles. I also would like to thank everyone at Elsevier for their help in putting this issue together. Mark Myerson has been a tremendous mentor and friend over the years and his tireless effort to educate and push the field of foot and ankle orthopedics to new horizons deserves our very special gratitude. My sincere appreciation to Mark Myerson for allowing me to participate in this issue and for his efforts in making this a very successful issue. I sincerely

Foot Ankle Clin N Am 18 (2013) xiii–xiv
http://dx.doi.org/10.1016/j.fcl.2013.08.009
1083-7515/13/$ – see front matter © 2013 Published by Elsevier Inc.

hope that you enjoy this edition and that the authors' efforts assist in the treatment of your patients.

Anish Raj Kadakia, MD
Department of Orthopedic Surgery
Northwestern University - Feinberg School of Medicine
Northwestern Memorial Hospital
675 North St. Clair Street, Suite 1350
Chicago, IL 60026, USA

E-mail address:
kadak259@gmail.com

Clinical and Radiographic Evaluation of the Cavus Foot

Surgical Implications

Anthony Perera, MBChB, FRCS(Orth)*, Abhijit Guha, MBChB, FRCS(Orth)

KEYWORDS

- Deformity • Radiological evaluation • Hindfoot alignment • Pes cavus • Cavovarus

KEY POINTS

- Clinical examination is the key to identifying deformity and functional loss.
- Plain radiographs are used for procedure selection and quantifying the correction required; the hindfoot alignment view is the best method of defining the degree of hindfoot varus.
- Magnetic resonance imaging scanning is used for assessing the peroneal tendons.
- Computed tomography is useful for 3-dimensional evaluation of the bony architecture, and single-photon emission computed tomography is useful for diagnosing areas of degeneration.

The term cavus foot has been rather loosely used to include a wide spectrum of foot shapes that have a high arch deformity in common. The arch may be high for a number of reasons, including high calcaneal pitch, excessive plantar flexion of the forefoot, or increased flexion in the midfoot. In many cases, there may be a torsional component responsible for or contributing to the high arch. There is varus of the hindfoot and varus and adduction of the forefoot also. The cavus foot has been traditionally associated with neuromuscular conditions like Charcot-Marie-tooth (CMT) disease, but a subtle form has been increasingly reported in the recent literature. The cavus foot is reported to be present in between 20% and 25% of the population.[1]

PLAIN FILM RADIOLOGY
Diagnosis of Pes Cavus

The cavus foot is defined on the lateral view as a calcaneal pitch angle (between the inferior surface of the calcaneum and the floor) of greater than 30° and Meary's angle (between the long axes of the talus and first metatarasal) of greater than 5°, although the average in most cavovarus feet approaches 20°. The normal calcaneum is at 5°

University Hospital of Wales and Spire Cardiff Hospital, 18 Melbourne Road, Llanishen, Cardiff CF145NH, UK
* Corresponding author.
E-mail address: FOOTANDANKLESURGERY@GMAIL.COM

Foot Ankle Clin N Am 18 (2013) 619–628
http://dx.doi.org/10.1016/j.fcl.2013.08.010
1083-7515/13/$ – see front matter © 2013 Elsevier Inc. All rights reserved.

valgus to the ankle, but it swings into varus in pes cavus, the magnitude reflecting the severity of the deformity (**Fig. 1**).

Ankle Radiographs

When weight-bearing radiographs of the ankle are obtained (**Fig. 2**), it is helpful to request the foot and ankle be shown on 1 view in order to get a feel for the overall deformity pattern. The lateral view may show the fibula sitting more posteriorly than usual; this demonstrates the external rotation deformity of the ankle that can occur in the distal tibia in severe cases. This can distort the view of the ankle and can be compensated for by internally rotating the ankle when taking the lateral view. This external rotation rarely requires correction fortunately, as this would involve a complex derotation osteotomy.

On the lateral view, the talus appears to be flattened, and there may be a double shadow; this reflects the rotation of the talus in the coronal and sagittal planes. As a result of these changes, it can be difficult to evaluate the joint space to evaluate the ankle for degeneration, although this is usually somewhat more obvious on the anteroposterior view. The sinus tarsi can often appear to be widened on the lateral view, and frequently the rotation and tilting of the talus produces a tarsal canal view. As a result, subtalar degeneration can be difficult to evaluate, and additional scans or joint injections may be required. However, lateral pain is common, and this may be due to lateral overload caused by the rigid hindfoot varus but may also be due to lax lateral ankle ligaments resulting in abnormal loading or peroneal tendon pathology. This additional soft tissue pathology is a critical factor that has significant bearing on the outcome of surgery evaluation; therefore a magnetic resonance imaging (MRI) scan should be ordered if there is any concern.

The ankle radiographs may show arthritic changes with narrowing and osteophyte formation of the tibiotalar joint, and this can be localized or generalized. If this is limited to the medial compartment of the ankle, then this may be amenable to rebalancing of the ankle with distal realignment with a possible additional proximal realignment (tibial osteotomy). If it is generalized, then the ankle must be addressed with either fusion or replacement. In all cases, the deformity of the foot must be corrected to neutralize the weight-bearing forces in the ankle and foot. If the foot deformity is not addressed, persistent lateral foot pain will be present (fusion), or ankle varus will recur (arthroplasty).

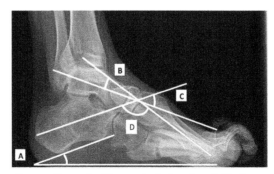

Fig. 1. Lateral standing radiograph. The posteriorly placed fibula and the talar double shadow are indicative of the rotation and talar tilt. Note the fifth metatarsal stress fracture that has failed to heal. (A) Calcaneal pitch angle greater than 30° in the cavus foot. (B) Talo first metatarsal angle, also known as Meary's angle, normal = 0° to 5°. (C) Talocalcaneal angle normally 35° to 50°; it is less than 35° in the cavovarus hindfoot. (D) First metatarsal calcaneal angle, also known as Hibb's angle, normal less than or equal to 45°.

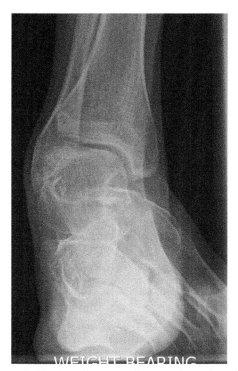

Fig. 2. AP ankle radiograph. The Standing x-ray does not show the talar instability that was evident when a true AP of the ankle was obtained using fluoroscopy and screening.

The ankle can be surprisingly mobile and comfortable even in the presence of marked radiographic changes, which emphasizes the need to correlate the radiographic appearance with the clinical symptoms prior to creating a surgical plan. If the ankle is symptomatic, but if the symptoms are mild or absent, then reconstruction of the foot deformity with rebalancing of the joint forces may be sufficient; this is the author's preferred surgical approach. However, if there are large osteophytes, particularly medially, these will be removed, as the alteration in the ankle mechanics that follows the reconstruction may result in the osteophytes producing an increased dorsiflexion block or becoming more painful. The gastrocnemius must also be assessed once the foot is realigned and any anterior tibiotalar osteophytes have been removed.

If the talus is tilted in varus on the AP ankle view, this finding implies the lateral ligament complex is incompetent, and it is likely that the deltoid ligament is reciprocally tight. This must alert one to the possibility that forefoot and hindfoot correction alone may be insufficient and that lateral ligament reconstruction may be required. Furthermore, it may not be possible to get the ankle neutral without a subperiosteal release of the deltoid ligament. One should be alert to the fact that in severe cases the peroneal tendons may be severely diseased and that they may not be sufficient for use in stabilization procedures. MRI or ultrasound can be helpful in determining the integrity of the tendons, allowing one to plan for use of the hamstring or allograft instead.

When contemplating lateral ligament reconstruction in these patients it is important to be aware of degeneration in the ankle. Irwin and colleagues[1] demonstrated that although good pain relief and stability can be achieved with lateral ligament reconstruction and foot osteotomy in those with moderate-to-severe degeneration, approximately one-third of patients do poorly, and the majority showed progression of their arthritis or required fusion. Therefore consideration should be given to definitive management of the degeneration in this group, although it is notable that even in the group with mild or no preoperative degeneration this was seen to develop in some cases. Appropriate patient counseling is important when performing reconstruction in the setting of known ankle arthritis. The patient must be aware that despite attempts to avoid arthroplasty or fusion, there is a significant rate of failure, and further surgery may be required in the future.

Foot Radiographs

Weight-bearing radiographs of the foot are also necessary (**Fig. 3**). Assessment of the first metatarsal alignment is helpful in evaluating the deforming drive coming from it and also for planning the surgical correction. If the talo first metatarsal angle (Meary's angle) is markedly increased, then the first metatarsal is severely plantarflexed, and it is likely that there will be significant pressure overload as a consequence. In this case, there is likely to be very little passive correctability, and a classic plantar fascia release and Jones procedure will be insufficient; dorsiflexing osteotomy will required. Even with this procedure, there is a limit to the amount of dorsal correction that can be achieved, and a multiple midfoot osteotomy or triple arthrodesis may be the only way of achieving an adequate correction by completely releasing the talonavicular joint capsule and derotating it fully.

It is important to pay attention to the plantarflexed first ray and achieve a full correction in those with anteromedial ankle degeneration as it forces the talus in dorsiflexion,

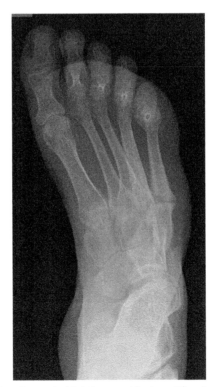

Fig. 3. DP Standing foot radiograph. Metatarsus adductus with external rotation of the talus.

causing anteromedial impingement. If the first ray is plantarflexed in isolation, then this can be addressed in isolation. However, when the metatarsals appear stacked on the lateral standing view, this suggests that that there is a differential metatarsal equinus responsible for the forefoot pronation, and thus the metatarsal correction needs to vary accordingly with different degrees of dorsiflexion correction. This can be achieved by removing less bone as one moves laterally from the first metatarsal to the second and third metatarsal. The fourth and fifth metatarsals rarely require dorsiflexion osteotomy. The final decision is made intraoperatively based on simulated weight-bearing. Therefore, in advanced cases in which it is necessary to address a marked forefoot overload, and the lesser metatarsals need to be corrected, the degree of correction must reflect this. The degree can be assessed clinically intraoperatively by palpation of the metatarsal heads. There is a limit to the amount of dorsal bone that can be removed from the lesser metatarsals in order to achieve a dorsal elevation. Fortunately, the first ray generally needs the biggest correction, with reducing amounts as one proceeds laterally. This therefore requires careful planning, and excision of an inverted trapezoid can be very useful in achieving shortening and dorsal elevation when a significant correction is required; this is best fixed with plating, as it is inherently unstable. Intraoperative palpation of the metatarsal heads is the most useful tool to determining the degree of correction required.

Lateral overload is a worrying sign in the presence of a fifth metatarsal stress fracture. The fifth metatarsal fracture has a low probability of union unless the lateral foot overload is corrected. If the deformity is driven by the first metatarsal alone, then this can be corrected in isolation. However, a calcaneal osteotomy may be required once a stress fracture has developed to significantly relieve the stress along the fifth metatarsal. Although this may be seen as a dramatic step, especially in an athlete, the deforming forces should be neutralized. When the cavovarus is mild to moderate, it is reasonable to attempt primary fixation of the stress fracture in isolation in conjunction with orthotic management. However, if the metatarsals appear to be markedly stacked and there is a severe hindfoot varus, then a lateralizing, closing wedge calcaneal osteotomy with ligament reconstruction as required is necessary. Dorsiflexion osteotomy of the first metatarsal is routinely performed in conjunction to eliminate any residual cavus and prevent recurrent varus. If the foot corrects with the Coleman block test, then the first metatarsal may be corrected in isolation, but this is uncommon in these patients.

If the toes are chronically dislocated in the presence of severe forefoot equinus, this is a very difficult situation. Wound healing problems, recurrence, and vascular insufficiency can all occur. This cannot be corrected by distal metatarsal osteotomy in the way that one generally manages this problem. It is likely that the skin, soft tissue, and vessels have never reached their full adult potential and thus have no hope of being sufficient to sustain a correction. Moreover there is in fact very little dorsal correction that can be performed through a distal correction. In this case, metatarsal head excision may be the most sensible option; occasionally even amputation of the toes may be safer.

A basal Barouk Rippstein Tourne (BRT)-type osteotomy allows for a greater degree of correction, but it is still limited; fixation can also be an issue. A basal BRT-type osteotomy does not allow for a shortening, however, thus a proximally performed shortening osteotomy removing an inverted trapezoid of bone with plate fixation may be utilized. The dorsoplantar (DP) and lateral radiographs can be used to plan the shortening to the neutral point (ie just proximal to the base of the toes). On the DP, it is usual to see to metatarsus adductus, and the metatarsals may appear narrowed as a consequence. However, this is not necessarily caused by a primary metatarsus adductus, as a cavovarus hindfoot and midfoot with forefoot pronation will always give this appearance. This is difficult to assess, and even CT scan is not helpful. However, an estimate of the degree of adductus can be evaluated using the deformity of the Talo first metatarsal angle on the DP view and subtracting the amount of heel varus on the hindfoot view, as this reflects the degree of true metatarsus adductus that is present. This can be signif-icant in severe cases, and especially in treated congenital talipes equinovarus. It is important to evaluate whether this is an apparent deformity caused by the forefoot pro-nation or whether it is caused by a primary issue at the talonavicular joint. In this case, or indeed even if it just very severe, the only way to correct it fully is via a triple arthrodesis.

Plain radiographs are helpful for getting a feel for the drivers of the deformity, as these vary from patient to patient; the diagnosis of the underlying etiology, however, and, most importantly, the function of the foot, rely on clinical examination. Plain film radi-ology is most useful for surgical planning, especially determining the site and magnitude of osteotomies or fusion. Identification of the apex of the deformity allows one to select whether to fuse or perform an osteotomy. If, for instance, the apex is at the navicular cuneiform or first tarsometatarsal joint, and the deformity is severe and fixed, it is the author's preference to perform a fusion, as there is a significant potential for correction at these sites.

Hindfoot Alignment Radiographs

Weight-bearing views that show tibia, talus, and calcaneum are essential. They were described originally by Cobey[2]; however, Saltzman and colleagues[3] have presented a modification of this technique that gives excellent reliability ($r = 0.97$). The patient stands on a radiolucent platform. The radiograph cassette is held at 20° from the ver-tical. A lead strip is placed at the posterior most extent of the foot perpendicular to its long axis in order to identify the horizontal plane. The radiograph tube is angled perpendicular to the cassette. The beam is centered at the level of the ankle, and the exposure includes the midtibia and below the calcaneus (**Fig. 4**).

However, just as importantly, Saltman and colleagues were able to produce norma-tive data that allow comparison of the preoperative status and thus surgical planning of the correction. As tibial rotation is part of the deformity, concern has been raised about the role of rotation in exaggerating the apparent varus.[4] Although the ankle rotates externally, the tibia itself has an internal rotation deformity. The most reliable way to assess this is with a CT scan performed at the level of the knee and the ankle. However, in the author's experience, it is rarely necessary for correction of this to be performed.

Evaluation of the hindfoot varus tilt is important, as its correction plays a key role in the surgical management of the cavovarus foot with regard to hindfoot instability and

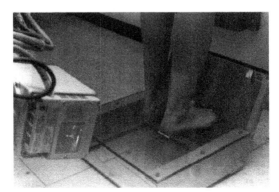

Fig. 4. The hindfoot alignment view. (*From* Saltzman CL, el-Khoury GY. The hindfoot alignment view. Foot Ankle Int 1995;16:572–6; with permission.)

forefoot overload. If the talus is tilted in the mortise, there is increased point loading. If this is associated with localized degeneration, then it may be improved by load redistribution with a lateralizing osteotomy and cheilectomy, even without lateral ligament stabilization.[5] Failures have been associated with a persistent talar tilt, instability, and a more widespread degeneration. In cases with normal ankle ligaments and persistent talar tilt despite realignment osteotomy, a shortening fibula osteotomy and deltoid ligament release can be considered. More recently, Krause and colleagues[5] have also shown that ankle degeneration in the presence of a horizontal ankle joint line and a cavovarus foot can be managed successfully with realignment of the heel.

The aim of the surgical plan is to aim for the ground reaction force to run just lateral to the center of the tibia; this evens out pressure distribution in the ankle and protects weak lateral tissues. If the deformity is above the talus, then supramalleolar osteotomy may be considered, and the weight-bearing AP ankle view is used to plan the osteotomy. This is best used in situations in which the varus tilt is due to deformity of the entire distal metaphysis resulting in a varus ankle joint with parallel joint surfaces rather than those cases in which there is localised tibial plafond loss resulting in a varus tilt of the talus though the body of the metaphysis remains parallel to the ground. A lateral closing wedge tibial osteotomy and shortening fibula osteotomy can be performed and are more reliable than an intra-articular opening wedge osteotomy. This latter technique can be used when there is a localized depression in the medial tibia; the distal extent of osteotomy ends in the subchondral bone at the lateral extent of this depression.

This weight-bearing view demonstrates alignment during midstance. It does not tell if the ankle is passively correctable, and it may be that the hindfoot is fixed or that there are correctable issues such as medial gutter osteophytes or a tight deltoid ligament that can be addressed without having to resort to fusion. It is possible to combine the hindfoot alignment view with a Coleman block test to assess correctability.

Screening of the ankle under fluoroscopy is helpful in preoperative planning and assessment of the ligaments; it is possible that the lateral ligament is worse than demonstrated on the plain films. Several authors have shown that realignment of the ground reaction force with calcaneal and metatarsal osteotomy can stabilize the ankle without ligament reconstruction. In the author's experience, if stabilization is required, this is done via a Chrisman-Snook type reconstruction with a slip of the peroneal brevis if it is intact or hamstring graft if not. If the talus is tilted and does not correct to neutral on screening, a bony correction is required. Occasionally this can be achieved by subperiosteal deltoid ligament release and debridement if the fibula is hypertrophied or a shortening osteotomy if it is normal.

Intraoperative screening after correction has been completed is invaluable. The issue with intraoperative screening is that it is a nonweight-bearing situation. Min and colleagues[6] have attempted to circumvent this by using a mortise view intraoperatively. They showed a mortise view taken intraoperatively (either prone or supine) with gentle plantar pressure with a mallet can be used to assess the position of the medial process of the posterior calcaneal tuberosity relative to the axis of the tibia. If the medial process is medial to this line, then the heel is in varus. This is helpful in determining the degree of correction achieved after a calcaneal osteotomy and negates any effect of tibial rotation on the appearance of deformity.

DEGENERATIVE JOINT DISEASE

Successful management of degenerative joint disease mandates that every joint that is contributing to the clinical symptoms is identified; otherwise postoperative pain may continue. However, it is preferable to fuse the minimum number of joints possible in order to maintain as much function as possible (unless these joints need to fused, because the deformity is severe and fixed). It can be difficult to make this decision based on clinical findings and even plain radiography. Diagnostic intra-articular anesthetic injections have been the mainstay of evaluation and are reliable.[7] However, it is important to utilize radio-opaque dye also, not just to confirm entry into the desired joint but also to look for communication between joints that may have a shared capsule, as this is common in the midfoot and even hindfoot and can confuse the picture if it is not known considered (**Fig. 5**).

To date, CT scan has been the mainstay of assessment of the presence of degeneration as well as defining the anatomy. More recently, single photon-emission computed tomography (SPECT) bone scans combined with CT (SPECT- CT) have been used increasingly in the foot and ankle. This technique builds on the more basic approach of simple bone scanning, which produces a generalized hotspot in the region of degeneration. With this refinement, it is possible to be specific about the site and severity of the degeneration. The images produced are also 3-dimensional, which further enhances the degree of localization that is possible. Pagenstert and colleagues[8] demonstrated the utility of this technique, particularly in areas in which the number and configuration of joints is complex (eg, the talonavicular and tarsometatarsal joints). This is particularly true in coronal plane hindfoot deformities,[9] in which it is possible to differentiate between global and isolated degeneration within the ankle joint with the clear implications this has for decision making on whether to fuse or realign. Krause and colleagues[10] have used an MRI protocol for quantification of ankle arthritis in pes cavovarus. They showed that it is possible to differentiate medial and lateral compartment wear. However, this area needs further evaluation and work on the clinical implications of these findings.

In the midfoot, it is common to see degenerative changes on the plain radiographs, but these appearances do not correlate well with the presence of symptoms; additionally, these techniques can be powerful in planning the scope of any midfoot fusion that is required. However, in the author's experience, MRI is less helpful in delineating the scope of degeneration. The appearance of edema does not appear to correlate with clinical symptoms, and joint injections with radio-opaque dye are the preferred method.

PERONEAL TENDON EVALUATION

The peroneal tendons play a crucial role in the etiology of the cavovarus phenotype, with relative weakness or paralysis of one or both. However, they can also suffer as a consequence of the posture of the hindfoot and more importantly as a consequence of instability if present. Thus it is not uncommon to find patients presenting with lateral ankle pain and swelling caused by peroneal tendinopathy and tearing. In some situations, the clinical diagnosis of peroneal pathology can be difficult; this is particularly true in the patient with recurrent instability who may well have one or more of a number of other pathologies (eg, a varus hindfoot, lateral ligament or capsular injury, distal fibula/lateral gutter impingement, or ankle or subtalar degeneration). Sometimes the lateral ankle can be bulky due to a large deformed distal fibula.

There is little written on peroneal imaging in pes cavus; however, in general the evaluation of tendinopathy appears to be best with MRI[11] and subluxation with ultrasound. The peroneal tendons pose a unique problem for MRI, as they change direction during their course. Thus the magic angle effect (MAE), which returns a bright signal in otherwise healthy tendons, cannot be compensated for with foot positioning.[12] The specific

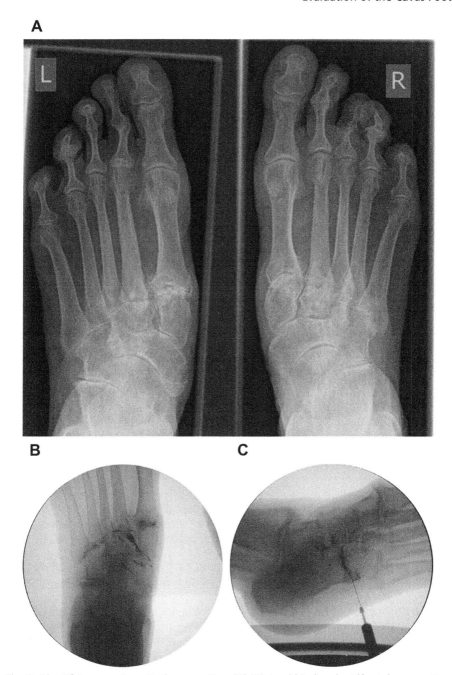

Fig. 5. Identifying symptomatic degeneration. (*A*) Bilateral hind and midfoot degeneration on plain films (taken from a pes planus case). (*B*) Left foot; despite the widespread appearances of degeneration, the pain in this foot entirely settled with a TMT injection, suggestive that the radiological evident hindfoot degeneration is not clinically relevant. However, note the widespread communication between the midfoot joints (needle in situ on the radiograph). (*C*) Right foot; calcaneocuboid injection fully resolved the hindfoot pain entirely. However, note the communication with the subtalar joint and thus it cannot be known whether the calcaneocuboid joint or the subtalar joint or both are responsible for the pain from this investigation alone.

evaluation and set up of MRI is not within the remit of this article other than to state that this requires an experienced musculoskeletal radiologist to set up and interpret the imaging; this topic is covered in detail by Schubert.[11]

However, one must be aware that the accuracy of even MRI in peroneal tendinopathy is limited. The specificity for diagnosing frank tears of the peroneus longus and brevis approached 100%, but the sensitivity was only 50%; the ability to pick up swelling in the brevis was poorer still.[13] Therefore a negative report must be taken with great caution.

SUMMARY

Plain film radiographs are essential in preoperative planning, not only to identify the deformity in order to select the appropriate procedure, but also to quantify the degree of correction that is required. The hindfoot alignment view allows one to urately measure the hindfoot varus, and intraoperative calcaneal axial views allow assessment of that correction. MRI and CT/SPECT CT have a major role in diagnosing certain secondary pathologies that are otherwise difficult to investigate. Clinical examination, however, is the key to successful management of pes cavus.

REFERENCES

1. Irwin TA, Anderson RB, Davis WH, et al. Effect of ankle arthritis on clinical outcome of lateral ankle ligament reconstruction in cavovarus feet. Foot Ankle Int 2010;31(1):941–8.
2. Cobey JC. Posterior roentgenogram of the foot. Clin Orthop Relat Res 1976;118: 202–7.
3. Saltzman CL, el-Khoury GY. The hindfoot alignment view. Foot Ankle Int 1995; 16(9):572–6.
4. Johnson JE, Lamdan R, Granberry WF, et al. Hindfoot coronal alignment: a modified radiographic method. Foot Ankle Int 1999;20(12):818–25.
5. Krause FG, Henning J, Pfander G, et al. Cavovarus foot realingment to treat anteromedial ankle arthrosis. Foot Ankle Int 2013;34(1):54–64.
6. Min W, Sanders R. The use of the mortise view of the ankle to determine hindfoot alignment: technique tip. Foot Ankle Int 2010;31(9):823–7.
7. Khoury NJ, el-Khoury GY, Saltzman CL, et al. Intraarticular foot and ankle injections to identify source of pain before arthrodesis. Am J Roentgenol 1996; 167(3):669–73.
8. Pagenstert GI, Barg A, Rasch H, et al. SPECT-CT imaging in degenerative joint disease of the foot and ankle. J Bone Joint Surg Br 2009;91(9):1191–6.
9. Knupp M, Pagenstert GI, Barg A, et al. SPECT-CT compared with conventional imaging modalities for the assessment of the varus and valgus malaligned hindfoot. J Orthop Res 2009;27(1):1461–6.
10. Krause FG, Klammer G, Benneker LM, et al. Biochemical T2 *MR quantification of ankle arthrosis in pes cavovarus. J Orthop Res 2010;28(12):1562–8.
11. Schubert R. MRI of peroneal tedinopathies resulting from trauma or overuse. Br J Radiol 2013;86(1021):20110750.
12. Mengiardi B, Pfirrmann CW, Schottle PB, et al. Magic angle effect in MR imaging of ankle tendons: influence of foot positioning on prevalence and site in asymptomatic subjects and cadaveric tendons. Eur J Radiol 2006;16(10):2197–206.
13. Park HJ, Lee SY, Park NH, et al. Accuracy of MR findings in characterizing peroneal tendon disorders in comparison with surgery. Acta Radiol 2012;53(7): 795–801.

The Idiopathic Cavus Foot–Not So Subtle After All

Ali Abbasian, FRCS (Tr & Orth)[a],*, Gregory Pomeroy, MD[b]

KEYWORDS

- Cavovarus deformity • Subtle cavus foot • Idiopathic

KEY POINTS

- Diagnosis of idiopathic cavus is subjective and requires careful clinical assessment.
- A multitude of symptoms have been associated with this foot shape.
- Nonsurgical treatment form the main stay of therapy unless symptoms are refractory to these measures.
- Treatment should be directed at correcting the underlying biomechanics as well as any associated symptoms.

INTRODUCTION

Pes cavus or cavovarus deformity has been long associated with neurologic disease resulting in a characteristic deformity. Conditions such as polio or hereditary sensori-motor neuropathy can lead to imbalance of lower limb muscle groups that have been long recognized to cause the typical cavovarus deformity and subsequent symptoms. Over the last 10 years, however, a mild variation of the cavovarus deformity has been increasingly accepted to exist without an identifiable underlying neurologic deficit. This mild variation may represent the "cavus end" of the normal distribution curve for arch height and is associated with a specific set of symptoms and complaints. This foot shape has been referred to as the subtle, nonneurologic, or idiopathic cavus and is becoming more readily identified as the source of a multitude of symptoms in the foot and ankle surgical practice.

Manoli and Graham[1] coined the term "Subtle cavus foot," which has since become increasingly used for the idiopathic form of the condition. Interestingly on searching the literature before this article, there had been no publications with the words Subtle and Cavus in the title or the abstract in the preceding 2 decades, while since this

The authors have nothing to disclose.
[a] Guy's and St Thomas' Hospitals NHS Foundation Trust, London SE1 7EH, UK; [b] Department of Mercy Hospital, University of New England, Portland, ME 04101, USA
* Corresponding author.
E-mail address: aabbassian@gmail.com

article, there have been 8 such publications. Manoli and Graham have not been alone in recognizing the deformity in its idiopathic form and previous authors[2,3] have appreciated that a proportion of patients presenting with symptoms relating to a cavovarus deformity do not have an underlying neurologic diagnosis.

It is true that, as one's awareness of the condition increases with experience, more cases will be observed. This was the case after the description of the "too many toes sign" for adult-acquired flat foot by Johnson and Strom.[4] What may seem subtle at first can become more obvious over time. Unfortunately, there are no reliable clinical signs or tests that can diagnose the condition objectively. The diagnosis is subjective and associated with a large interobserver variation.

In this article an up-to-date account of the clinical and radiological diagnosis as well as the surgical and nonsurgical management of the idiopathic cavus foot are described.

PATHOANATOMY

Cases of secondary or neurologic cavovarus deformity can arise from a multitude of factors resulting in the final deformity. Some have divided the deformity into posterior, anterior, or mixed cavus.[5] The posterior cavus or calcaneocavus is characterized by a high calcaneal pitch of greater than 30°. An angle greater than 30° is formed between the inferior border of the calcaneus and the ground on the weight-bearing lateral radiograph. It is generally seen in conditions where there is a weakness of the gastrocsoleus complex leading to a calcaneus deformity of the hindfoot, typically seen in the cavus foot secondary to conditions such as poliomyelitis or after a cerebrovascular accident, and is not a typical feature of the subtle cavus foot. In contrast, anterior cavus is secondary to plantar flexion of the forefoot, can be associated with metatarsus adductus, and is the usual finding in idiopathic (subtle) cavus. The first ray is normally at a greater inclination than the lesser rays but this can vary depending on the severity of the deformity. In the subtle cavus foot the deformity is often mild and clawing of the toes is absent or mild.

The exact cause in the cavus foot has been subject to debate and both the intrinsic[6,7] and the extrinsic[2,3] muscle imbalances may play a role in the final deformity. Price and colleagues[7] examined a pediatric population with an underlying neuropathy and demonstrated an earlier and more severe involvement of the intrinsic muscles of the foot as compared with the extrinsic muscles with degeneration occurring in lumbricals and the interossei, inherently resulting in an "intrinsic-minus" foot and subsequent claw deformity of the toes. The relatively rare occurrence of marked clawing in idiopathic and subtle types of cavus may suggest a more extrinsic cause in this condition.

An imbalance between the antagonistic muscles and in particular peroneus longus and tibialis anterior is often listed as a cause.[3] An interesting study[2] analyzed the morphology of 5 lower leg muscles from 17 patients with forefoot pes cavus with those of normal muscles. Of the 17 cases, only 8 had an identifiable underlying neurologic diagnosis. In the idiopathic cases they demonstrated both histologic and magnetic resonance imaging (MRI) evidence of peroneus longus enlargement. They concluded that, in idiopathic forefoot pes cavus, fiber hypertrophy in peroneus longus (relative to tibialis anterior) may contribute to the cavus deformity. This so-called "peroneus longus overdrive" results in plantar flexion of the first ray. Because of the tripod effect of the foot, this will result in a varus hindfoot position.[3,8] In the normal foot in early stance the Chopart joints (talonavicular and calcaneocuboid) are locked and the hindfoot is in varus, which is the case at heel strike. However, as the ground reaction force moves distally, the hindfoot tilts into valgus, unlocking the Chopart joints, which requires pronation of the midfoot. In the cavus foot because of the plantar flexed posture of the first ray, the midfoot remains supinated, which prevents the unlocking of the Chopart joints, resulting in a hindfoot varus position for much of the stance phase and leading to a stiff foot with high pressures over the lateral side. The flexibility of the hindfoot in the normal foot acts as a shock absorber. This shock absorption is much reduced in the cavus foot.

Another key pathoanatomical property of the subtle cavus foot is the ubiquitous presence of an isolated gastrocnemius contracture.[1] The exact reason for the coexistence of the 2 conditions is not clear but patients with cavus feet often have tight calves with isolated gastrocnemius tightness. This isolated gastrocnemius tightness has several deleterious effects: first, it increases the plantar pressures in the forefoot and the plantar fascia, resulting in symptoms. In addition, because of the varus position of heel and the medial position of the Achilles insertion, it also acts as a deforming hindfoot inverting force, which worsens the problem. It has also been suggested[1] that the relative equinus position of the ankle secondary to gastrocnemius tightness can place the vector pull of peroneus longus (relative to tibialis anterior) at a greater mechanical advantage, thus enhancing its first ray plantar flexion effect.

SYMPTOMATOLOGY

The subtle cavus foot can present with a whole array of symptoms affecting the entire lower limb and may coexist at the time of presentation or the patient may describe the presence of these in their past. **Box 1** lists the symptoms associated with cavus deformity, some which deserve a more detailed mention and have been described in the following sections.

Forefoot

Patients often present with symptoms relating to forefoot overload. Forefoot overload is due to a combination of gastrocnemius tightness and the cavus deformity. Lesser metatarsalgia is a common complaint. If the underlying cavus is not appreciated, it is easy to misdiagnose. Many patients present who have had multiple neuroma excisions followed by "stump neuroma" excisions from adjacent web spaces in the same foot to cure their forefoot pain. This pain was due to an underlying undiagnosed cavus deformity. The problem is often confused further by the presence of an enlarged nerve on ultrasound examination. Ultrasound imaging of a neuroma, however, has been shown to overdiagnose neuromata even in experienced hands.[9] In this study more than half of the asymptomatic control subjects had an enlarged nerve on ultrasonic examination. It is not clear what the incidence of asymptomatic enlarged interdigital nerves is in cavus feet compared with the general population, but one can postulate that excessive weight-bearing stress on the forefoot, which is known to result in neuromas,[10] may play a significant role. Misdiagnosing Morton's neuromata in those with cavus feet may therefore be a common occurrence.

Overload of the first metatarsal head and the sesamoids can lead to pain or even fracture of the sesamoids. Disorders of the sesamoids are difficult to manage in this group of patients and local surgery on the sesamoids may be futile without the correction of the underlying equinus or cavus deformity.

Midfoot

Stress fractures of the lesser metatarsals especially in the athletic subgroup can exist. Fractures of the fifth metatarsal are common. These stress fractures can present after

---

Box 1
Conditions associated with the subtle cavus foot

Metatarsalgia

Metatarsal stress fractures

Sesamoiditis

Sesamoid fractures

Fracture and/or nonunion of the fifth metatarsal base

Tarsometatarsal arthrosis

Nonspecific arch pain

Peroneus longus/brevis tendinopathy and/or tears

Peroneal tendon subluxation or dislocation

Os peroneum syndrome

Enlarged peroneal tubercle

Low-lying peroneus brevis muscle belly

Recurrent ankle sprains or instability

Anteromedial ankle impingement

Plantar fasciitis or plantar fascia tears

Isolated gastrocnemius contracture

Achilles insertional and noninsertional tendinopathy

Haglund syndrome

Stress fractures of tibia

Vertical sheer stress fracture of the medial malleolus

Medial tibial stress syndrome and shin splints

Varus ankle arthrosis

Varus malposition of ankle arthroplasty

Medial knee compartment disorders (eg, arthrosis or meniscal tears)

Iliotibial band syndrome

External tibial torsion

---

relatively minor trauma and would have a tendency for nonunion. In the authors' experience, it is not uncommon to receive a tertiary referral for help in the management of a patient with a nonunion of a fifth metatarsal fracture, sometimes after attempts at internal fixation has failed, only to realize that an underlying idiopathic cavus has been overlooked. Even after successful radiological union, those with an underlying cavovarus foot may continue to complain of pain over the fifth metatarsal. This pain is of course secondary to the mechanical overload and not due to the fracture and is more likely to respond to realignment by orthotics or through surgery. Lateral midfoot or hindfoot overload can present with laterally based pain. This overload can lead to high signals in various bones on MRI and lead the unsuspecting surgeon to entertain nonspecific diagnoses such as cuboid syndrome. It is interesting that in one study[11] an association between lateral ankle sprains and cuboid syndrome was identified. It is recognized that laterally based foot pain and ankle sprains can coexist in subtle cavus feet.[1,12] It would have been interesting to note if the patients in that study had this underlying pathologic abnormality in the first place.

Hindfoot

The symptoms are primarily from reduced shock absorption and gastrocnemius tightness in the hindfoot and may include Achilles pathologic abnormality or plantar fasciitis. The varus position of the heel may lead to a prominence of the posterior superior calcaneal tuberosity laterally and therefore those with an already enlarged Haglund process are more likely to develop retrocalcaneal bursitis or Haglund syndrome. Although in a study looking at the association between insertional Achilles tendonitis and a high calcaneal pitch of the cavus foot shape, a statistically significant difference was found; this was thought to be clinically insignificant because the difference was just 2° of inclination.[13]

Ankle

Ankle instability and recurrent sprains are common presenting symptoms.[12] These patients often have pain over the lateral ligamentous complex and may have failed a previous attempt at surgical repair (Brostrom or modified Brostrom ligament repair). Again, it is important to identify the underlying cavus if further intervention is to be successful. Peroneal tendon symptoms may include tendinopathy, tears, subluxations, or dislocations. It is not uncommon to find a hypertrophied and low-lying muscle belly of the peroneus brevis at surgery, although an association has not been described. Anteromedial impingement between talar and tibial spurs has been described in the athletic population and is also thought to be more common in those with subtle cavus feet.[14] Longstanding varus overload and recurrent sprains can also obviously lead to secondary osteochondral lesions and arthrosis in the medial half of the ankle joint.

Lower Limb

The inefficient shock absorption and the medially displaced mechanical axis of the lower limb result in excessive medial compressive and lateral tensile forces, resulting in medial tibial stress syndrome or tibial stress fractures, especially in runners. In the knee it can predispose to medial compartment pathologic abnormality and iliotibial band friction syndrome.

CLINICAL ASSESSMENT

The clinical examination of the foot should begin with the evaluation of the patterns of wear affecting the patient's shoe. This evaluation is especially valuable in cases of subtle cavus where the deformity may be difficult to appreciate and is subjective. The authors have undertaken a blinded, prospective, case control study (Abbasian and Pomeroy, unpublished, 2012) evaluating the patterns of wear in the shoes of those with a clinical diagnosis of subtle cavus and observed a common wear pattern in a significant proportion (**Fig. 1**). The finding of this type of wear may give the clinician some objective evidence in the quest for diagnosis.

The aim in the clinical evaluation of the primary or idiopathic cavus foot is not only to confirm the presence of the condition but also to differentiate it from secondary and neurologic types and to identify any underlying neurologic disease. An evaluation of the entire lower limb is mandatory. Calf wasting or hypertrophy and the knee alignment should be noted.

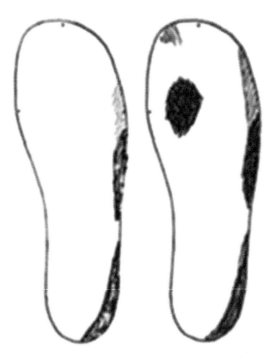

Fig. 1. Two common patterns of shoe wear seen in those with a subtle cavus foot.

Inspection

A vast amount of information can be obtained from mere observation of the weight-bearing posture of the foot. Some or all of the following may be present (**Fig. 2**):

- From the front:
  - Peek-a-boo heel
  - High arch
  - Metatarsus adductus or a "bean-shaped" foot
  - Prominence of the dorsolateral foot and the extensor digitorium brevis
  - Pronation of the hallux
  - Clawing of toes: marked deformity is suspicious of a neurologic etiology
- Sole of the foot:
  - Callosity under the first or fifth metatarsal heads
  - Thickening or callosities over the lateral border of the foot or base of the fifth metatarsal
- From the rear:
  - Varus heel: The medial position of the heel when compared with the midline of the calf
  - Prominence or posterior position of the lateral malleolus

It is important to standardize the patient's standing position. Patients are asked to stand with the feet at shoulder width apart to ensure the medial borders of the hallux of both feet are in parallel alignment, thus negating any effect the rotation of the lower limb may have on the appearance of the heel. In this position any appearance of the medial border of the heel, the so-called peek-a-boo heel,[1] is

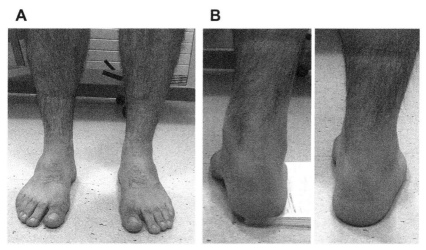

Fig. 2. Patient with bilateral subtle cavus deformity. (*A*) The peek-a-boo heels and the prominent extensor digitorium brevis muscle on the dorsolateral aspect of the foot seen on the frontal view and the varus posture of the heel on the rear view. (*B*) Correction of the varus on the Coleman block.

considered a sign of excessive heel varus. This excessive heel varus is then confirmed by looking from behind. After heel varus is confirmed, it is important to establish the flexibility of the hindfoot using the Coleman block test.[15] The Coleman block test differentiates a forefoot-driven varus, which is the expected finding in the primary idiopathic types from those caused by hindfoot pathologic abnormality (see **Fig. 2**). A stiff hindfoot may be due to tarsal coalition, subtalar arthrosis, previous fracture, or muscular spasm. Appropriate further investigation should then be undertaken.

Several conditions may mask or mimic the presence of a varus heel and should be looked out for if a false positive or negative diagnosis is to be avoided (**Table 1**).

Examination

Other than examination of the specific area of the presenting complaint, for example, performing an anterior drawer test or talar eversion stress tests for those presenting

Table 1 Conditions resulting in false positive (+ve) or negative (−ve) diagnosis of varus		
	Condition	**Explanation**
+VE	Morbid obesity	Inability to stand on the medial border of foot because of large bulky thighs
	Painful hallux or first Metatarsophalangeal joint	Protective supination
	Painful plantar fasciitis	Protective supination to avoid standing on the medial insertion of plantar fascia
	Displaced heel pad	Medial prominence without true varus
−VE	Metatarsus adductus	Masking heel varus
	Medial ankle swelling	Masking heel varus

with recurrent ankle stability, the following additional maneuvers are performed in all patients:

- Coleman block test (see **Fig. 2**)
- Silfverskoild test: To assess the presence of an isolated gastrocnemius tightness, this test is performed by comparing the range of ankle dorsiflexion with the knee in flexion and in extension. Various authors use different range of dorsiflexion as cut-off for diagnosis.[16,17] The authors diagnose gastrocnemius tightness if the foot cannot be made plantigrade (ie, remains in equinus) with the knee in full extension.
- Subtalar range of motion: It is important to note that patients with varus heels lack much subtalar eversion, which is particularly important when, for example, the standing position of the heel is in neutral alignment but the patient is unable to achieve any further eversion. This means that the standing (neutral) position represents the maximal valgus position of the hindfoot and thus lateral overload and varus are likely to occur during gait.
- Neurologic examination: A full assessment should be undertaken to detect any muscular imbalance. All muscle groups but particularly the Peroneus longus and brevis as well as tibialis posterior and anterior should be examined for power and graded from 1 to 5 on the Medical Research Council grading system. An assessment of any sensory deficit is made and, if neurologic disease is suspected, a full neurologic examination of both the upper and the lower limbs must be completed.
- Spine: A gross inspection of the spine to detect any evidence of spinal dysraphism, for example patches of midline hair or nevus, can be a useful adjunct if a neurologic cause is suspected.

RADIOLOGY AND SPECIAL INVESTIGATIONS

The authors use plain weight-bearing radiographs of the foot and ankle as the workhorse of the assessment in this condition and most patients rarely need any other investigations. Although a wide variation is seen, the following radiological features can help in considering the diagnosis:

- Lateral weight-bearing radiograph of foot and ankle (**Fig. 3**)
  - Plantar flexed first metatarsal (a positive Meary angle[18]). Meary angle is the angle between a line drawn along the axis of the first metatarsal and that of the talus and is normally at $0 \pm 5°$.
  - Stacked metatarsals: The first and medial metatarsals tend to be at a greater inclination, while the lateral metatarsals are more in contact with the ground, which gives a stacking effect where the metatarsals can be seen separately with a lesser amount of overlap than in a normal situation.
  - High arch: Medial cuneiform to fifth metatarsal base distance is increased as compared with normal.
  - Subtalar view: The subtalar joint on the true lateral view will have the appearance similar or approaching that seen on a subtalar or a Broden view because of the inversion of the hindfoot.
  - Posterior position of fibula: Due to the varus hindfoot position and the inevitable external rotation of the lower limb, the fibula will appear more posterior to the tibia than in the normal situation.
  - Increased calcaneal pitch (normal 10–20°).
  - Thickening or fractures of the base of the fifth metatarsal due to mechanical overload.

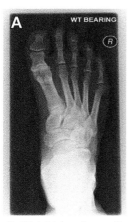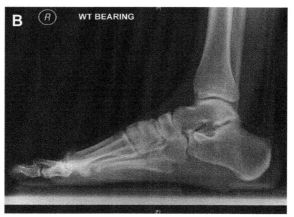

Fig. 3. Weight-bearing radiographs of a patient with a subtle cavus deformity.

- Dorsoplantar weight-bearing radiograph of foot (see **Fig. 3**)
  - Metatarsus adductus
  - Hypertrophy or stress fractures of the lesser metatarsals
  - Talonavicular over coverage: Much of the reverse of that described for the acquired adult flat foot[19]
  - Reduction of the talocalcaneal angle: The angle of the long axis of talus and calcaneus on the dorsoplantar view decreases (getting close to zero) as they become parallel (normal value greater than 25°).
- Anteroposterior weight-bearing view of the ankle
  - Height of the ankle from the floor to top of the talar dome is increased.
- Special views can be performed for further evaluation:
  - Hindfoot alignment view[20] or the long-axial view[21] can be helpful in confirming the varus position of the calcaneal contact point and is occasionally useful
  - Oblique views can help in evaluating the individual metatarsals in cases of fracture and are useful when a calcaneonavicular coalition[22] or when anteromedial impingement from a medial talar neck osteophyte[14] is suspected.
- Computed tomographic scans are helpful to assess the hindfoot joints for evidence of arthrosis, look for tarsal coalition, and rule out the presence of a fracture or large talar osteochondral lesions and may occasionally be indicated.
- MRI scans are on the whole used for identification of any associated conditions, such as tendinopathy, ligament insufficiency, or chondral lesions, especially of the talus. However, most of their findings can be clinically detected and in our practice are not frequently used when managing patients with idiopathic cavus.
- Neurologic investigations are best performed by a neurologist and preferably one with an interest in peripheral neuropathies. If an underlying neurologic disease is suspected (**Box 2**), the authors' practice is to seek a neurologic consult. Electromyography, nerve conduction studies, imaging of the entire spine and brain, biopsy, or genetics testing may be necessary in some cases.

MANAGEMENT
Nonsurgical

A large number of patients with milder symptoms associated with a cavus deformity can be treated successfully with conservative and nonsurgical means. The

---

Box 2
Features suggestive of an underlying neurologic etiology

Family history of peripheral neuropathy

Family history of claw toes or cavus foot

History of rapid onset and progression of cavus deformity

Unilateral disease or marked difference in severity between the 2 sides

Severe deformity especially one that is associated with marked clawing of the toes and hallux

Lateral and anterior compartment wasting in the lower leg (inverted champagne bottle legs)

Neurologic findings on examination

Neurologic findings or symptoms in the hands or upper limbs

Spinal dysraphism

---

conservative measures should focus on the associated pathologic abnormality as well as the underlying cavus deformity.

Nonsurgical treatment of the associated condition

Attention should be paid to the presenting symptom and the conservative strategy would depend on this. For example, those with ankle instability are treated with proprioception training and an ankle supportive brace, especially worn during exercise. The treatment of those with a fractured fifth metatarsal base may be a walking boot or even a cast and patients with Achilles tendonosis may benefit from eccentric stretching of the tendon.[23]

Nonsurgical treatment of the underlying cavus

The focus in nonsurgical treatment of the underlying cavus is to realign the hindfoot correctly to offload the lateral border of the foot (orthotics) and to overcome the gastrocnemius tightness (calf stretching).

The ideal orthotic for the subtle cavus foot[24] aims to tilt the hindfoot out of varus which is achieved through the following characteristics of the in-shoe orthotic:

- Full length
- Minimal or absent medial arch support
- Lateral hindfoot to midfoot wedge
- Recessed first ray

The amount of wedging or recess can be tailored to the severity of the deformity. 'Off the shelf' and prefabricated orthotics are also available that may be suitable for milder deformity (**Fig. 4**).

It is a common mistake by running shops to advise those with a cavus foot to purchase shoes with a high arch support. In the authors' experience, this happens frequently and leads to worsening of the symptoms as the medial arch support acts to further tilt the foot in supination and the hindfoot in varus.

SURGERY

When nonsurgical measures fail to control the symptoms, surgery may be indicated. The following surgical algorithm[25] was used:

- Correction of equines: It is imperative that the equinus deformity is addressed first. The Silfverskiold test was repeated intraoperatively. If a global

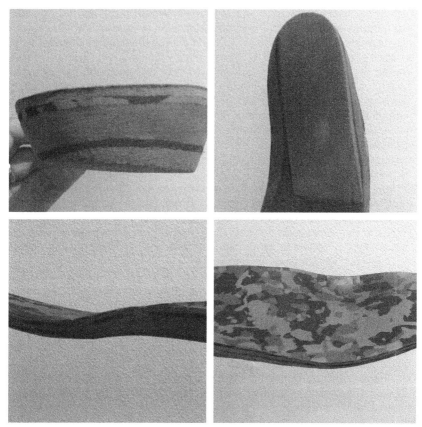

Fig. 4. A bespoke orthotics. The lateral heel wedge presents throughout the hindfoot and midfoot (top 2 images), the very low arch, and the recess for the plantar flexed first ray (*bottom right and left images, respectively*).

gastroc-soleus contracture was present, a tendoachilles lengthening using a triple hemisection is performed. Most cases however will present with an isolated gastrocnemius tightness. This tightness is addressed using a gastrocnemius recession[26] in a modification of the Strayer technique. The Strayer technique is a posteromedial approach through the gastroc-soleus interval. The sural nerve is protected and the gastrocnemius aponeurosis is released from medial to lateral.

- Dorsiflexion osteotomy of first metatarsal: Dorsiflexion osteotomy is performed next if the preoperative Coleman block test has confirmed a forefoot-driven pathologic abnormality (see **Fig. 2**). A longitudinal dorsal incision is made over the first tarsometatarsal joint and while the extensor hallucis longus tendon is protected, a dorsal closing wedge osteotomy is performed with a saw at a point 10 mm from the first tarsometatarsal joint. The osteotomy is closed and fixed using a lag screw of 3.5 mm diameter from dorsal and distal (metatarsal shaft) to proximal and plantar (metatarsal base). A burr is used at the entry point to aid buttress and to countersink the head of the screw.
- Correction of hindfoot varus: In cases where Coleman block test does not fully correct the hindfoot varus or there is residual varus after the dorsiflexion

osteotomy, a calcaneal osteotomy is often performed in addition to a dorsiflexion first metatarsal osteotomy. The skin incision is an oblique incision in line with the planned osteotomy at around 45° to the floor. The tuberosity is then displaced in a lateral direction by about 5 to 10 mm until the hindfoot is in neutral or in a slight degree of valgus. While an assistant holds the displacement, the surgeon secures it with 1- or 2-part threaded 6.5-mm screws and the final position is checked on orthogonal fluoroscopy images. Although there is some concern regarding postoperative iatrogenic tarsal tunnel syndrome following a lateral shift calcaneal osteotomy, in the authors' experience, a prophylactic release is not necessary.

- Peroneus longus (PL) to brevis (PB) tendon transfer: Although several different tendon transfers have been successfully used in cavovarus reconstruction, the authors' preferred transfer in cases of subtle cavus is the PL to PB transfer. If, after the correction of hindfoot varus and equinus there was no residual first ray plantar flexion, no further procedure is performed.[25] However if the first ray is plantar flexed beyond the lesser rays, then a PL to PB transfer is undertaken. The authors' threshold for performing this transfer is further lowered if a coexisting peroneal tendinopathy is present. In this situation the PB is often more involved with multiple tears. A complete excision of PB and transfer via a PL graft is then performed. A curvilinear incision is performed 1 cm proximal and posterior to the tip of the fibula extending to the interval between PB and PL. While care is taken not to disrupt the superior peroneal retinaculum , the PL and PB are transferred in a side-to-side manner before transecting the PL distal to the transfer and thus removing the peroneal overdrive on the first ray. If the SPR is taken down, the authors do this by subperiosteal dissection from the fibula and repairs it via suture anchors at the completion of the tendon transfer. The authors have not encountered any secondary deficits long term in patients undergoing this procedure for nonneurologic cavus.

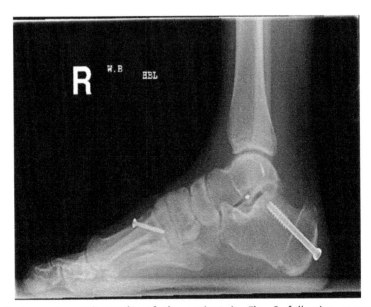

Fig. 5. Postoperative radiographs of the patient in **Fig. 3** following a cavus foot reconstruction.

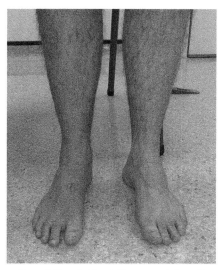

Fig. 6. Patient after correction of the right subtle cavus deformity who had presented with recurrent instability. Note the asymptomatic uncorrected left subtle cavus foot.

- Associated surgical procedures are then performed. These surgical procedures are frequently a Brostrom ligament repair or internal fixation of a fifth metatarsal fracture.
- Postoperatively the patients are placed in a bulky Jones dressing with a posterior splint for 2 weeks followed by a further 6 weeks of casting and they remain non-weight-bearing during this time.

Fig. 5 demonstrates the postoperative radiographs of the patient in **Fig. 3**, with subtle cavus deformity, who presented with debilitating lateral right hindfoot pain and ankle instability. **Fig. 6** is the same patient 3 months after surgery to correct the right foot. Note the subtle cavus deformity of the asymptomatic left foot.

SUMMARY

Idiopathic cavus deformity even in its mild form can result in several associated symptoms. Management of these symptoms without addressing the underlying biomechanical abnormality may result in failure of treatment. A careful clinical assessment is paramount.

REFERENCES

1. Manoli A 2nd, Graham B. The subtle cavus foot, "the underpronator". Foot Ankle Int 2005;26(3):256–63.
2. Helliwell TR, Tynan M, Hayward M, et al. The pathology of the lower leg muscles in pure forefoot pes cavus. Acta Neuropathol 1995;89(6):552–9.
3. Mosca VS. The cavus foot. J Pediatr Orthop 2001;21(4):423–4.
4. Johnson KA, Strom DE. Tibialis posterior tendon dysfunction. Clin Orthop Relat Res 1989;239:196–206.
5. Japas LM. Surgical treatment of pes cavus by tarsal V-osteotomy. Preliminary report. J Bone Joint Surg Am 1968;50(5):927–44.

6. Mann RA, Missirian J. Pathophysiology of Charcot-Marie-Tooth disease. Clin Orthop Relat Res 1988;234:221–8.

7. Price AE, Maisel R, Drennan JC. Computed tomographic analysis of pes cavus. J Pediatr Orthop 1993;13(5):646–53.

8. Aminian A, Sangeorzan BJ. The anatomy of cavus foot deformity. Foot Ankle Clin 2008;13(2):191–8, v.

9. Symeonidis PD, Iselin LD, Simmons N, et al. Prevalence of interdigital nerve enlargements in an asymptomatic population. Foot Ankle Int 2012;33(7):543–7.

10. Wu KK. Morton's interdigital neuroma: a clinical review of its etiology, treatment, and results. J Foot Ankle Surg 1996;35(2):112–9 [discussion: 187–8].

11. Jennings J, Davies GJ. Treatment of cuboid syndrome secondary to lateral ankle sprains: a case series. J Orthop Sports Phys Ther 2005;35(7):409–15.

12. Chilvers M, Manoli A 2nd. The subtle cavus foot and association with ankle instability and lateral foot overload. Foot Ankle Clin 2008;13(2):315–24, vii.

13. Shibuya N, Thorud JC, Agarwal MR, et al. Is calcaneal inclination higher in patients with insertional achilles tendinosis? A case-controlled, cross-sectional study. J Foot Ankle Surg 2012;51(6):757–61.

14. Manoli A 2nd. Medial impingement of the ankle in athletes. Sports Health 2010;2(6):495–502.

15. Coleman SS, Chesnut WJ. A simple test for hindfoot flexibility in the cavovarus foot. Clin Orthop Relat Res 1977;123:60–2.

16. DiGiovanni CW, Kuo R, Tejwani N, et al. Isolated gastrocnemius tightness. J Bone Joint Surg Am 2002;84(6):962–70.

17. Abbassian A, Kohls-Gatzoulis J, Solan MC. Proximal medial gastrocnemius release in the treatment of recalcitrant plantar fasciitis. Foot Ankle Int 2012;33(1):14–9.

18. Meary R, Filipe G, Aubriot JH, et al. Functional study of a double arthrodesis of the foot. Rev Chir Orthop Reparatrice Appar Mot 1977;63(4):345–59 [in French].

19. Chadha H, Pomeroy G, Manoli A 2nd. Radiologic signs of unilateral pes planus. Foot Ankle Int 1997;18(9):603–4.

20. Saltzman CL, el-Khoury GY. The hindfoot alignment view. Foot Ankle Int 1995;16(9):572–6.

21. Reilingh ML, Beimers L, Tuijthof GJ, et al. Measuring hindfoot alignment radiographically: the long axial view is more reliable than the hindfoot alignment view. Skeletal Radiol 2010;39(11):1103–8.

22. Crim JR, Kjeldsberg KM. Radiographic diagnosis of tarsal coalition. AJR Am J Roentgenol 2004;182(2):323–8.

23. Ohberg L, Lorentzon R, Alfredson H. Eccentric training in patients with chronic Achilles tendinosis: normalised tendon structure and decreased thickness at follow up. Br J Sports Med 2004;38(1):8–11 [discussion: 11].

24. LoPiccolo M, Chilvers M, Graham B, et al. Effectiveness of the cavus foot orthosis. J Surg Orthop Adv 2010;19(3):166–9.

25. Maskill MP, Maskill JD, Pomeroy GC. Surgical management and treatment algorithm for the subtle cavovarus foot. Foot Ankle Int 2010;31(12):1057–63.

26. Abbasian A. Isolated contracture and gastrocnemius recession. Foot Ankle Int 2013;34(2):307–8.

Treatment of Ankle Instability with an Associated Cavus Deformity

Hilary A. Bosman, BSc, MBBS, MRCS (Eng), FRCS (Tr & Orth),
Andrew H.N. Robinson, BSc, MBBS, FRCS, FRCS (Orth)*

KEYWORDS

• Cavus • Varus • Foot • Ankle • Heel • Ligaments • Surgery • Orthosis

KEY POINTS

- Subtle cavovarus is common and can potentiate chronic ankle instability.
- Comprehensive examination of foot position is mandatory when assessing patients presenting with ankle pain and instability.
- The "peek-a-boo heel" sign is an indicator of subtle cavus.
- Nonsurgical management options include appropriate footwear, custom orthoses, and gastrocnemius stretching.
- Isolated lateral ligament repair is less likely to be successful in the presence of uncorrected cavovarus.
- Operative management includes correction of foot alignment. Ankle fusion may be required in late-stage instability with osteoarthritis.
- Ankle arthritis may occur following acute or chronic ligamentous injury. Early surgical correction of cavovarus with ankle instability has the potential to reduce progression.

INTRODUCTION

The ankle is the most commonly injured joint in sport and at work and the lateral ligament complex is the most frequently injured structure.[1] Studies in Norway and Finland have reported that ankle sprains account for between 16% and 21% of all athletic injuries.[2,3] An estimated 42,000 severe ankle sprains are sustained in the United Kingdom each year.[4] Basketball and soccer have high injury rates of 31% and 45%, respectively.[5,6] The vast majority of ankle sprains are treated nonoperatively but, unfortunately, not all recover. An estimated 30% to 40% will have chronic complaints following recurrent sprains.[7,8] Potential complications include persisting pain and

Conflicts of Interest: None declared.
Department of Trauma and Orthopaedics, Cambridge University Hospitals NHS Trust, Box 37, Hills Road, Cambridge CB2 2QQ, UK
* Corresponding author.
E-mail address: fredthefoot@virginmedia.com

Foot Ankle Clin N Am 18 (2013) 643–657
http://dx.doi.org/10.1016/j.fcl.2013.08.005
1083-7515/13/$ – see front matter © 2013 Elsevier Inc. All rights reserved.

foot.theclinics.com

instability secondary to ligamentous incompetence, peroneal tendon injury, synovitis, chondral damage, and end-stage osteoarthritis. Lateral ligament injuries are common and of significance, leading to career-ending injury in professional sportspersons, and difficulties at work with significant morbidity in the nonsporting population.

Abnormal foot shape adversely affects the biomechanics of the ankle and may predispose to the first and subsequent injuries. Although cavovarus is more common in ankle instability,[9,10] in a review article on the characteristics of people with recurrent ankle sprains, a high arch was not identified as a clear risk factor.[11] The Ontario Cohort Study and a study by Twellar and colleagues[12] also did not show any significant correlation between leg and foot alignment and the risk of injury.[13]

The aim of this article is to review the role of cavus in foot and ankle injury and to summarize the current strategies in the management of cavovarus foot associated with ankle instability.

PES CAVUS AND CAVOVARUS

Ledoux and colleagues[14] found an incidence of 24% pes cavus and 19% pes planus in their review of 2047 diabetic feet. Pes cavus (defined in **Box 1**) describes an increase in the height of the medial longitudinal arch of the foot, which does not flatten on weight bearing. Pure cavus causes few symptoms and rarely requires surgical treatment. The hindfoot alignment is the crucial factor in determining the foot type and likely development of symptoms. The association of cavus with heel varus overloads the lateral structures of the foot and ankle,[15] and may progress to end-stage disease with varus ankle arthritis.[16,17]

A plantarflexed first ray, forefoot pronation and adduction, and hindfoot varus are all components of the cavovarus foot. Hindfoot varus is described as being forefoot or hindfoot driven. In forefoot-driven varus, excessive plantarflexion of the first metatarsal leads to the hindfoot moving into varus, as opposed to simple varus malalignment of the heel in hindfoot-driven varus. The Coleman block test (see later discussion) is designed to differentiate between these two causes of hindfoot varus. The varus malalignment may, however, originate higher up, for example in a varus malunited tibial fracture.

Foot shape is likely to be normally distributed, from cavovarus at one extreme to planovalgus at the other. The causes of pes cavus are shown in **Box 2**. The hereditary sensory and motor neuropathies are the most commonly encountered causes of severe pes cavus in clinical practice, although approximately one-third are idiopathic.[18] Manoli describes the "subtle" cavovarus foot in detail elsewhere in this issue.

FOOT MECHANICS IN RELATION TO ANKLE INSTABILITY

A plantarflexed first ray prevents the normal hindfoot progression from varus into valgus in the stance phase of the gait cycle. In varus the hindfoot is locked, as the calcaneocuboid and talonavicular joints are divergent, whereas in valgus the joints are parallel, unlocking the hindfoot. The valgus/unlocked midtarsal joint is "supple" and

---

Box 1
Definition of pes cavus

pes: Latin for foot

cavus: Cavity or hollow

varus: Deviation of the distal segment of a limb toward the midline

---

Box 2
Causes of pes cavus

Neurologic

Hereditary sensorimotor neuropathy, myelodysplasia, Friedreich ataxia, cerebral palsy, poliomyelitis, spinal cord tumors, sciatic nerve tumors, muscular dystrophy, spinocerebellar degeneration, spinal muscular atrophy, syringomyelia, primary cerebellar disease, multiple sclerosis, Guillain-Barré syndrome, interstitial hypertrophic childhood neuritis, occult hydrocephalus

Traumatic

Postcompartment syndrome, fracture malunion, burn contracture

Residual congenital deformity

Including congenital talipes equino-varus, arthrogryposis multiplex congenita, tarsal coalition

Idiopathic

---

allows shock absorption, whereas the varus hindfoot is stiff. The loss of shock absorption results in potential stress injuries.[19] Hindfoot varus also increases the risk of damage to the lateral structures of the foot and ankle, as a consequence of both the reduced shock absorption and the increased load through the weaker lateral structures. Nevertheless, the effect of varus hindfoot alignment can cause symptoms throughout the lower limb. Manoli and Graham[20] list several problems associated with cavovarus (**Box 3**).

Strauss and colleagues[21] reviewed a cohort of 160 patients with chronic lateral ankle ligament instability. The associated pathology included peroneal tendon injuries in 28%, os trigonum symptoms in 13%, lateral gutter ossicles in 10%, and anterior tibial spurs in 3%; however, only 8% of these patients had hindfoot varus.

THE "SUBTLE CAVUS" FOOT

The "peek-a-boo" heel sign, first described by Manoli and colleagues[22] in 1993, is the clinical condition whereby the heel is visible on the medial side when viewing the patient from the front with the feet in neutral rotation (**Fig. 1**). Manoli considers mild cavovarus to be at one end of the binomial distribution of foot shape, in contrast to the significant abnormalities outlined in **Box 3**.[20] He believes that this subtle deformity is idiopathic, familial, and inherited by poorly delineated genetic determinants.

Manoli considers the primary deforming force to be the plantarflexed first metatarsal, which is thought to be a result of peroneus longus overdrive.[23–25] The first metatarsal becomes fixed in flexion. A vicious cycle is then entered into, as plantarflexion of the first ray and equinus deformity increase the plantarflexion vector of the peroneus longus, further flexing the first metatarsal. The dorsiflexion vector of the tibialis anterior is reduced, exacerbating the problem. A shortened gastrocnemius with more medial pull will cause further varus, as most patients with a subtle cavus foot have a tight gastrocnemius; this is a factor in speeding the development of the deformity. As a result, the presence of equinus can precipitate the progression of the cavus.[20,26,27]

RADIOLOGIC CORRELATION

Markers of cavus on a lateral radiograph include talar height, talocalcaneal angle, talometatarsal angle or Meary angle of greater than 20°, Hibb angle between the long axis

---

Box 3
Lower limb abnormality associated with cavovarus foot alignment (after Manoli)

Ankle instability

Subtalar instability

Os trigonum

Peroneal tendon tears and dislocation

Enlarged peroneal tubercle

Painful os peroneum syndrome

Enlarged distal fibula

Stress fracture base of fourth and fifth metatarsal

Calluses under first and fifth metatarsal heads

Sesamoid overload

Chondromalacia

Plantar fasciitis

Vertical stress fracture medial malleolus

Metatarsus adductus

Midfoot arthritis

Varus ankle arthritis

Medial compartment knee osteoarthritis

Iliotibial band friction syndrome

Tibia stress fracture

Exertional compartment syndrome

Tight gastrocnemius

---

of the calcaneum and first metatarsal of greater than 45°, and calcaneal pitch of greater than 30° (**Figs. 2–4**).[28] Louwerens and colleagues[29] studied 33 patients with chronic lateral ankle ligament instability. Although cavovarus deformity was commonly found on clinical examination, the investigators were unable to correlate this to

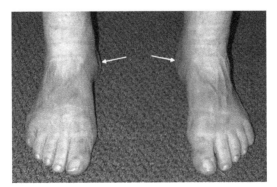

Fig. 1. Peek-a-boo heel. The patient is observed from the front. Ensure the feet are in neutral alignment. The medial contour of the heel is seen "peeking" into view from the front (*arrows*), in contrast to the more valgus heel, where it is not seen.

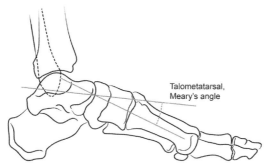

Fig. 2. A Meary or talometarsal angle (angle between long axis of talus and first metatarsal on weight-bearing lateral radiograph) of more than 20° is consistent with cavus.

radiologically measured foot geometry. Larsen and Angermann[9] compared 95 patients undergoing surgery for lateral ankle instability with a normal group and found the surgical group to have increased arch height on standing lateral radiographs.

The relationship between the varus heel of a cavus foot and chronic instability has been well documented.[30] A varus tibial plafond and a posteriorly placed fibula are also predisposing factors in chronic ankle instability.[31,32]

The mortise ankle radiograph is examined for ankle congruence and alignment. A modified Cobey view can be taken to measure hindfoot alignment while weight bearing.[33] Computed tomography (CT) may also be useful in determining hindfoot alignment and specific joint involvement. In a Canadian study, simulated weight-bearing CT scans showed patients with lateral ligament instability to have increased heel calcaneal varus in comparison with controls.[34]

NEUROMUSCULAR ISSUES IN CHRONIC INSTABILITY

Functional instability may be as important as the mechanical factors in chronic injury. Although subtle cavovarus is not considered to have a neurologic cause, it is likely that subclinical muscle imbalance is present in these patients. Recovery from an ankle sprain and joint protection is reliant on accurate proprioceptive and neuromuscular control.

"Closed-loop" control, or reactive ankle control, is diminished following lateral sprain in the normal ankle.[35] During everyday activities the foot and ankle position is

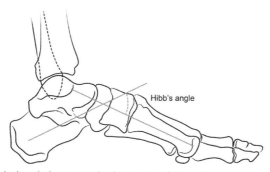

Fig. 3. A Hibb angle (angle between the long axis of the calcaneum and first metatarsal) of more than 45° indicates cavus.

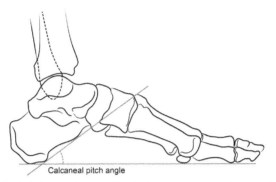

Calcaneal pitch angle

Fig. 4. A calcaneal pitch (angle between inferior calcaneal surface and ground) of more than 30° indicates cavus.

constantly adjusted to provide a stable base for propulsion. Afferent proprioceptive messages act on the muscles controlling the ankle position. In particular, peroneal muscle function is critical for dynamic ankle-joint control. Following ankle injury, not only is afferent proprioception impaired but the efferent peroneal muscle reaction times are reduced.[36] In a study of 21 patients with functional instability, patients were subjected to a 30° inversion surface "trap door" while walking, and peroneal activities were recorded electromyographically.[35] Alpha motor-neuron excitability was impaired in the affected ankles in those with functional instability. Peroneal muscle dysfunction is thought in part to be secondary to arthrogenic muscle inhibition as a result of swelling and joint effusion.

Preparatory or "open-loop" control is also impaired following acute sprain,[37,38] which affects the distal prepositioning and joint tension crucial for impact attenuation and load bearing. Peroneal muscle reflex response alone has been shown to be too slow to protect the ankle,[38] therefore impaired background joint-stabilization processes will increase the vulnerability of the ankle to repeated injury. In a gait-assessment study of 24 patients with functional instability, Delahunt and colleagues[37] showed changes in foot positioning during the swing phase as well as increased inversion before and at initial contact. The hindfoot varus in the cavovarus foot will therefore increase the likelihood of reinjury.

The theory of articular deafferentation secondary to direct injury of ligamentous proprioceptors and arthrogenic muscle inhibition is central to current rehabilitation principles following ankle sprain.[36,38] Although no studies have compared peroneal muscle reaction times or open-loop control measures in the cavovarus and the normal foot, it would not be unreasonable to expect greater sensorimotor dysfunction in the cavovarus foot, which would further impair dynamic control.

ASSESSMENT OF THE CAVUS FOOT

In assessing the patient with ankle instability (outlined in **Box 4**), it is important to consider the patient's foot shape. Failure to recognize a subtle cavovarus can result in the failure of surgery.[26,39] In a study of military patients treated for recurrent instability, hindfoot varus was present in 8%. The most common reason for failure of ligament reconstruction was failure to correct the hindfoot varus, which accounted for 28% of the patients with failed surgery.[21]

Examination should commence with the patient standing barefoot. Foot alignment and arch height should be recorded from the front and behind. The heel alignment

Box 4
Assessment of acute-on-chronic ankle instability

History

Traumatic ankle injury, single or recurrent

Footwear and orthoses

Sport

Exclude neuromuscular disease including familial

Examination

Joint line tenderness/synovitis

Ligamentous tenderness

Mechanical stability to varus/anterior draw/rotation

Heel alignment including "peek-a-boo" heel

Peroneus longus overdrive

Coleman block test

Silfverskiöld test

Neurologic examination

Imaging

Anteroposterior and lateral standing radiographs

Modified Cobey view

Ultrasonography (in particular for tendon abnormality)

Magnetic resonance imaging (to determine ligamentous involvement and/or chondral lesion)

Computed tomography (useful for assessment of bony details, such as osteochondral lesions and fractures)

Other

Examination under anesthetic

should be observed, paying particular attention to subtle varus, including the peek-a-boo heel sign (see **Fig. 1**). A normal hindfoot lies in 5° valgus. Proximal malalignment should also be excluded, whether varus/valgus or rotational. The lower back and entire lower limb should be examined and a comprehensive neurovascular examination carried out.

Walking aids and shoes, including the wear pattern, should be noted. The gait pattern should be viewed for any asymmetry. In particular, foot positioning at first contact and through the stance phase with excessive loading on the lateral border of the foot and heel. The Coleman block test should be performed to ascertain whether hindfoot varus is correctable (**Fig. 5**).

With the patient either seated or supine, areas of swelling or tenderness should be noted. The lateral ligaments and peroneal tendons should be palpated. The sole of the foot should be inspected for callosities or signs of overload; in the cavovarus foot it is not unusual to find marked callosities under the first and fifth metatarsal heads.

Passive and active range of movement of the ankle, hindfoot, and forefoot should be noted, and stability tested. Resistance to varus, rotation and anterior draw should be compared with that of the contralateral ankle. Although difficult to distinguish,

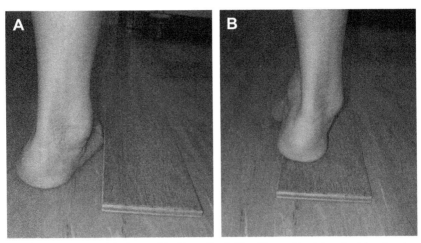

Fig. 5. (*A, B*) Coleman block test/hindfoot flexibility. The patient is asked to stand on a wooden block. The block most be positioned so that the first ray is unsupported. Correction of the hindfoot varus with the block in place confirms a mobile subtalar joint and forefoot-driven cavovarus.

variations in muscle balance should be tested with resisted inversion and eversion. The influence of peroneal overdrive is determined, as is gastrocnemius tightness established, using the Silfverskiöld test.

Peroneal overdrive is measured with the patient positioned supine with the knee extended. The examiner's thumbs are placed on the plantar aspect of the foot at the level of the metatarsal heads, one thumb medially under the first and the other under the lesser metatarsals. With the ankle in neutral, the patient is asked to plantarflex the foot against the examiner's resisting thumbs. A positive test is when the examiner's thumbs are pushed away with more force by the first metatarsal than the lateral forefoot. The foot plantarflexes into a pronated position.

The Silfverskiöld test assesses gastrocnemius tightness. With the patient positioned supine, with the knee extended and the talonavicular joint in neutral, the ankle is passively dorsiflexed. The test is repeated with the knee flexed to 90°. Knee flexion relaxes the gastrocnemius (which crosses the joint) but leaves soleus tension unaffected. A large increment in dorsiflexion with the knee flexed implies isolated gastrocnemius tightness. If ankle dorsiflexion with the knee extended is less than 5°, gastrocnemius contracture is diagnosed.[40] This aspect should be addressed at the time of surgery.

NONOPERATIVE TREATMENT

First-line treatment, particularly after an acute sprain, should be nonoperative with ankle-focused physiotherapy. A gastrocnemius-stretching program should be initiated to treat equinus.[26] Together with orthotic management, this may be sufficient to functionally stabilize the ankle. In a study of 93 patients with subtle cavovarus, a custom orthotic provided reduced pain scores and instability in 92%.[41] The type of orthotic chosen depends on the Coleman block test. When the hindfoot is supple, accommodation of the plantarflexed first ray will allow the hindfoot to correct. The metatarsal head should be recessed and the heel slightly elevated to allow for equinus, with lateral forefoot posting and a lowered arch support to accommodate correction. If the block test shows a hindfoot-driven cavus, a lateral heel wedge with first metatarsal recess is the appropriate orthosis.[19,26] In the authors' practice a laterally posted forefoot orthosis is most commonly used.

OPERATIVE TREATMENT

Operative treatment should only be considered in carefully selected patients. The individual's willingness to commit to a prolonged rehabilitation program should be ensured before embarking on surgical treatment. All aspects of the disorder need to be considered and dealt with at a single sitting where possible. The primary treatment goal is correction of foot shape, providing the most beneficial mechanical environment for ankle stability and function.

Surgical priorities are tailored to the individual and are dependent on foot shape. Corrective procedures may be considered in the following order.

Dorsiflexion First-Ray Osteotomy

The authors' preferred method is the BRT (Barouk, Rippstein, Toullec) osteotomy. In this procedure the first metatarsal is approached in the interval between the extensor hallucis longus and brevis tendons. The first metatarsal is exposed and a dorsal wedge is excised around 2 cm from the tarsometatarsal joint. The cut is angled plantarwards and posteriorly at approximately 60° to the longitudinal axis of the first metatarsal (**Fig. 6**). Care is taken to leave the plantar cortex intact. The osteotomy is then closed with upward pressure under the first metatarsal head, and sequential saw cuts are removed until the required dorsiflexion is achieved. The amount of dorsiflexion required varies, but should be palpating the level of the first and second metatarsal heads. It is usually necessary to take a wedge of between 3 and 5 mm from the dorsum of the first metatarsal. A headless, cannulated compression screw is then used to secure the osteotomy. It is important to place the guide wire for the screw at least 1 cm proximal to the osteotomy site to prevent splitting of the dorsal metatarsal cortex. In the majority of cases an isolated first metatarsal osteotomy can be undertaken. If there is excessive flexion of the second and third metatarsals, similar osteotomies of the lesser metatarsals may be carried out to balance the forefoot and prevent transfer lesions.

Heel Varus

A calcaneal osteotomy is undertaken through a short extended lateral approach.[42] The limbs of the incision are shortened to 6 cm, rather than the traditional 12 cm.

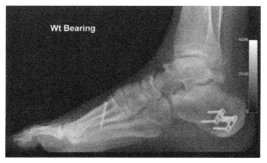

Fig. 6. Postoperative correction following first metatarsal dorsal osteotomy and calcaneal lateral translational osteotomy.

The calcaneum is osteotomized with an oscillating saw. The authors believe that a translational osteotomy rather than a lateral closing wedge of the os calcis realigns the mechanical axis more effectively. This osteotomy is fixed using a calcaneal locking step plates and a 10-mm translation is optimal. Calcaneal osteotomy reduces the contact stresses in cadaveric ankles.[43]

Lateral Ligament Reconstruction

In the majority of cases a Brøstrøm repair with the Gould modification is used. Through a linear incision over the distal fibula, the lateral ankle ligaments are exposed. The extensor retinaculum is carefully dissected free and the anterior talofibular and calcaneofibular ligaments are mobilized subperiosteally off the fibula. The ligaments are then tightened and reattached to the fibula with a #2 Ethibond suture using drill holes through the distal fibula. The extensor retinaculum is then reefed over the ligamentous repair. The importance of the retinacular tightening is two-fold; first, it provides strength and second, as the extensor retinaculum crosses the subtalar joint it stabilizes the subtalar joint.

If there is complete absence of the ligamentous complex, the authors use a modified Chrismann-Snook procedure. The peroneus brevis tendon is split and harvested percutaneously. The tendon is then passed through a drill hole in the distal fibula and secured to the calcaneum with an interference screw. If the peroneus brevis tendon is torn and unsuitable for a lateral ankle ligament reconstruction, a free hamstring graft is used. This procedure requires consideration preoperatively to allow proper consent, and also preparation of the limb.

Gastrocnemius Lengthening

The authors undertake a gastrocnemius-soleus lengthening through a 4-cm longitudinal, midline incision, usually with the patient supine and the assistant holding the leg elevated. The incision is made just distal to the musculotendinous junction in the calf. Care is taken to avoid the sural nerve. The musculotendinous junction is isolated and the tendinous portion divided across its full width.

ASSOCIATED PATHOLOGY

It is important to correct associated abnormalities. The authors routinely undertake an ankle arthroscopy to allow debridement of chondral lesions and anterior ankle synovitis if necessary.

The peroneal tendons are explored at the time of the lateral ligament repair, using the Krause classification for treatment of peroneus brevis tendon tears.[44] Debridement and repair are recommended for tendons that have damage to less than 50% of their cross-sectional area. Excision of the damaged segment and tenodesis to the peroneus longus are recommended for tendons with destruction of greater than 50% of the cross-sectional area. For patients in whom the peroneus longus is a driver of the cavus foot, the tendon is transected distal to the tenodesis, defunctioning the peroneus longus.[44,45]

On occasion a Jones fracture may require fixation, in which case a 5-mm cannulated screw is inserted percutaneously.

Where there is an underlying neurologic cause, tendon transfers may also be appropriate. Such a procedure will be highly dependent on the individual's deficit and residual function, and is beyond the scope of this article.

Postoperatively the patient is placed in a well-padded below-knee back-slab plaster with the foot and ankle in neutral dorsiflexion for 2 weeks. At this stage the patient is transferred into a full cast or removable boot for a further 4 to 6 weeks. After removal of the plaster cast, an intensive rehabilitation program is commenced. Once full range of movement has been achieved, strength and proprioception are focused upon, with the aim of returning to linear running at 4 months and full sport at 6 months.

CONSEQUENCES OF CHRONIC INSTABILITY

Ligamentous instability predisposes to ankle osteoarthritis. Valderrabano and colleagues[46] showed ligamentous ankle injury to be the primary cause in 7% of a cohort of patients with established ankle arthritis. The latent period for the development of ankle arthritis was 34 years. A cadaveric study has shown the cavovarus foot to be associated with increased anteromedial ankle-joint pressure.[47] Thus the cavovarus foot is at increased risk of osteoarthritis, even in the absence of traumatic injury, although repeated episodes of instability will exacerbate posttraumatic changes.

The development of ankle arthritis in the ankle with varus instability raises two issues. First, does correction of the instability prevent development of the arthritis? This point is moot, as there is no definitive evidence. However, it would seem sensible to assume that reducing the incidence of traumatic sprains will reduce the incidence of intra-articular damage to the ankle.

Second, and perhaps more pertinently, how and when does one treat the patient with varus ankle instability and ankle arthritis with reconstruction as opposed to fusion or replacement? In a small series of patients, Fortin and colleagues[17] advocated cavovarus correction in moderate ankle arthritis and ankle fusion in grade III arthritis where there is joint-space obliteration. Emphasis in both cases was on correction of the varus; all patients had good resolution of their preoperative symptoms.

There remains some controversy as to the most effective surgical method for treating late instability in the presence of mild to moderate degeneration. Beals and Manoli[48] achieved good results on undertaking an isolated first metatarsal dorsiflexion osteotomy in a series of 4 elderly patients with advanced forefoot-driven ankle instability with equinus. Irwin and colleagues[49] reported on 22 patients in whom cavovarus deformity was treated with a calcaneal osteotomy with or without first metatarsal osteotomy and lateral ankle ligament reconstruction. The results were better in patients without joint-space narrowing. "A cautious and realistic approach" to patients with joint-space narrowing was recommended.

Krause and colleagues[45] reported improvements in AOFAS (American Orthopaedic Foot and Ankle Society) hindfoot scores in 11 of 13 patients in whom realignment surgery was performed for the treatment of anteromedial ankle arthrosis. The realignment of the cavovarus was aggressive, including calcaneal, fibular, and first metatarsal osteotomies, peroneus longus to brevis tendon transfer, and lateralization of the tibialis anterior insertion. Of note, lateral ankle ligament reconstruction was omitted from their surgical regime. It was found that if the varus of the ankle was corrected the outcome was good, even in the presence of joint-space narrowing.

Takakura's group[50,51] has reported 2 series of patients with varus malalignment of the tibial plafond treated with fibular osteotomy and an opening-wedge supramalleolar tibial osteotomy. The lateral ankle ligaments were not repaired. In these 2 series durable relief of the symptoms is reported with a follow-up of 8 years. All patient groups did well, except those with complete obliteration of the joint space between the tibial plafond and talar dome. The group with degeneration localized to the space between the medial malleolus and the medial aspect of the talus also did well. Takakura recommends overcorrection of the deformity, but considers malalignment of the distal tibial plafond to be associated with the Japanese habit of sitting cross-legged, which in Western practice is a rare form of malalignment.

Knupp and colleagues[52] reported good results using extensive surgery with supramalleolar tibial combined osteotomy with correction of the foot shape using calcaneal osteotomy with or without midfoot osteotomy or arthrodesis and lateral ankle ligament repair. These investigators conclude that the main risk factors for failure in supramalleolar osteotomy are osseous imbalance (eg, noncorrection of the fibula), ligamentous insufficiency, and ankles with intra-articular varus arthritis.

In the authors' experience, treatment of the cavovarus foot with ankle arthritis requires judgment in the selection of cases, and is technically demanding. The presence of complete loss of joint space on a standing radiograph mitigates a good result, as does failure to achieve correction on the postoperative standing radiograph. All aspects of the deformity should be corrected. An arthroscopic debridement of the ankle is undertaken, as is a calcaneal osteotomy, first metatarsal dorsiflexion osteotomy, and tendon rebalancing if required. The authors repair the lateral ankle ligament complex and debride any peroneal tendon tears; nevertheless, it is the correction of the foot shape and reestablishment of ankle congruence that is the most important factor in determining outcome. Improving ankle-joint mechanics will improve the patient's symptoms by offloading the area of damaged chondral surface, normalizing contact stresses and stability. When arthrosis is severe with a preserved subtalar joint, ankle fusion with alignment correction at the level of the ankle is preferred. Combined ankle and subtalar joint fusion using a transcalcaneal nail is considered if there is significant degeneration at both joints. If the malalignment is supramalleolar, for example in a malunited tibia, a supramalleolar osteotomy is undertaken (**Figs. 7** and **8**).

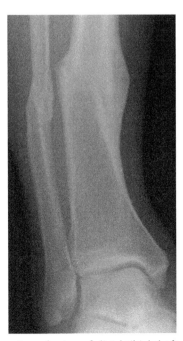

Fig. 7. Ankle varus secondary to malunion of distal tibial shaft.

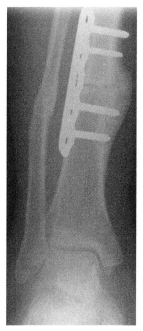

Fig. 8. Postoperative correction following valgus osteotomy.

SUMMARY

A cavovarus foot is a frequently encountered but underestimated cause of chronic ankle instability. A high index of clinical suspicion for abnormal foot shape and biomechanics should be maintained when treating patients with ankle instability. Management of ankle instability in the presence of cavovarus must address the malalignment. Correction of foot shape should be combined with formal ligamentous repair. Appropriate rehabilitation and sensorimotor retraining should be included in all treatment programs. Without restoration of joint-protective function, osteoarthritis is not uncommon.

REFERENCES

1. Mafulli N, Giuseppe Longo U, Petrillo S, et al. Lateral ankle instability. Orthop Trauma 2012;26:20–4.
2. Maehlum S, Daljord OA. Acute sports injuries in Oslo: a one year study. Br J Sports Med 1984;18:181–5.
3. Sandelin J. Acute sports injuries: a clinical and epidemiological study [dissertation]. Helsinki (Finland): University of Helsinki; 1988. p. 1–66.
4. Bridgman SA, Clement D, Downing A, et al. Population based epidemiology of ankle sprains attending accident and emergency units in the West Midlands of England, and a survey of UK practice for severe ankle sprains. Emerg Med J 2003;20:508–10.
5. Ekstrand D, Tropp H. The incidence of ankle sprains in soccer. Foot Ankle Int 1990;11:41–4.
6. Greene TA, Shillman SK. Comparison of support provided by a semi-rigid orthosis and adhesive ankle taping before, during, and after exercise. Am J Sports Med 1990;18:498–506.

7. Konradsen L. Seven-year follow-up after ankle inversion trauma. Scand J Med Sci Sports 2002;12:129–35.
8. Van Rijn RM, Van Os AG, Bernsen RM. What is the clinical course of acute ankle sprain? A systematic literature review. Am J Med 2008;121:324–31.
9. Larsen E, Angermann P. Association of ankle instability and foot deformity. Acta Orthop Scand 1990;61:136–9.
10. Rose KJ, Hiller CE, Mandarakas M, et al. SP20 Predictors of ankle instability in children and young people with Charcot-Marie Tooth disease. Neuromuscul Disord 2012;22:892.
11. Hiller C, Nightingale EJ, Lin CC, et al. Characteristics of people with recurrent ankle sprains: a systematic review with meta-analysis. Br J Sports Med 2011; 45:660–72.
12. Twellar M, Verstappen FT, Huson A, et al. Physical characteristics as risk factors for sports injuries: a four-year prospective study. Int J Sports Med 1997;18: 66–71.
13. Walter SD, Hart LE, McIntosh JM, et al. The Ontario Cohort Study of running related injuries. Arch Intern Med 1989;149:2561–4.
14. Ledoux WR, Shofer JV, Ahroni JH, et al. Biomechanical differences among pes cavus, neutrally aligned and pes planus features subjects with diabetes. Foot Ankle Int 2003;24:845–50.
15. Klaue K. Hindfoot issues in the treatment of the cavovarus foot. Foot Ankle Clin 2008;13:221–7.
16. McBride D, Ramamurthy C. Chronic ankle instability: management of chronic lateral dysfunction and the varus tibiotalar joint. Foot Ankle Clin 2006;11:607–23.
17. Fortin PT, Guettler JH, Manoli A. Idiopathic cavovarus foot and lateral ankle instability: recognition and treatment implications relating to ankle arthritis. Foot Ankle Int 2002;23:1031–7.
18. Brewerton DA, Sandifer PH, Sweetnam DR. "Idiopathic" pes cavus: an investigation into its aetiology. Br Med J 1963;14:659–61.
19. Chilvers M, Manoli A. Subtle cavus foot and association with ankle instability and lateral foot overload. Foot Ankle Clin 2008;13(2):315–524.
20. Manoli A, Graham B. The subtle cavus foot, 'the underpronator', a review. Foot Ankle Int 2005;26:256–63.
21. Strauss JE, Forsberg JA, Lippert FG. Chronic lateral ankle instability and associated conditions: a rationale for treatment. Foot Ankle Int 2007;28:1041–4.
22. Manoli A, Smith DG, Hansen ST Jr. Scarred muscle excision for the treatment of established ischemic contracture of a lower extremity. Clin Orthop 1993;292: 309–14.
23. Krause FG, Wing K. Neuromuscular issues in cavovarus feet. Foot Ankle Clin 2008;13:245–58.
24. Mosca VS. The cavus foot. J Pediatr Orthop 2001;21:423–4.
25. Vienne P, Schoniger R, Helmy N, et al. Hindfoot instability in cavovarus instability: static and dynamic balancing. Foot Ankle Int 2007;28:96–102.
26. Desai SN, Grierson R, Manoli A. The cavus foot in athletes: fundamentals of examination and treatment. Oper Tech Sports Med 2010;18:27–33.
27. Solis G, Hennessy MS, Saxby TS. Pes cavus: a review. Foot Ankle Surg 2000;6: 145–53.
28. Aminian A, Sangeorzan BJ. The anatomy of cavus foot deformity. Foot Ankle Clin 2008;13:191–8.
29. Louwerens JW, Ginai AZ, VanLinge B, et al. Chronic instability of the foot and foot geometry: a radiographic study. The Foot 1996;6:13–8.

30. Myerson M. Current therapy in foot and ankle surgery. St Louis (MO): Mosby Yearbook; 1993. p. 203–9.
31. Sugimoto K, Samoto N, Takura Y, et al. Varus tilt of the tibial plafond as a factor in chronic ligament instability of the ankle. Foot Ankle Int 1997;18:402–5.
32. Scranton PE, McDermott JE, Rogers JV. The relationship between chronic ankle instability and variations in mortise anatomy and impingement spurs. Foot Ankle Int 2000;21:657–64.
33. Saltzman CL, El-Khoury GY. Hindfoot alignment view. Foot Ankle Int 1995;16: 572–6.
34. Van Bergeyk AB, Younger A, Carson B. CT analysis of hindfoot alignment in chronic lateral ankle instability. Foot Ankle Int 2001;23:37–42.
35. Palmieri-Smith R, Hopkins JT, Brown TN. Peroneal activation deficits in persons with functional ankle instability. Am J Sports Med 2009;37:982–8.
36. Hertel J. Sensorimotor deficits with ankle sprains and chronic ankle instability. Clin Sports Med 2008;27:353–70.
37. Delahunt E, Monaghan K, Caulfield B. Altered neuromuscular control and ankle joint kinematics during walking in subjects with functional instability of the ankle joint. Am J Sports Med 2006;34:1970–6.
38. Gutierrez GM, Kaminski TW, Douex AT. Neuromuscular control and ankle instability. PM R 2009;1:359–65.
39. Ortiz C, Wagner E. Cavovarus foot reconstruction. Foot Ankle Clin 2009;14: 471–87.
40. DiGiovanni CW, Kuo R, Tejwani N, et al. Isolated gastrocnemius tightness. J Bone Joint Surg Am 2002;84:962–70.
41. LoPiccolo M, Chilvers M, Graham B, et al. Effectiveness of the cavus foot orthosis. J Surg Orthop Adv 2010;19:166–9.
42. Freeman BC, Duff S, Allen PE, et al. The extended lateral approach to the hindfoot. J Bone Joint Surg Br 1998;80:139–42.
43. Steffensmeier SJ, Saltzman CL, Berbaum KS, et al. Effects of medial and lateral displacement calcaneal osteotomies on tibiotalar joint contact stresses. J Orthop Res 1996;14:980–5.
44. Krause JO, Brodsky JW. Peroneus brevis tendon tears: pathophysiology, surgical reconstruction and clinical results. Foot Ankle Int 1998;19:271–9.
45. Krause FG, Henning J, Pfander G, et al. Cavovarus foot realignment to treat anteromedial ankle arthrosis. Foot Ankle Int 2013;34:54–64.
46. Valderrabano V, Hinterman B, Horisberger M, et al. Ligamentous post-traumatic ankle osteoarthritis. Am J Sports Med 2006;34:612–20.
47. Krause F, Windolf M, Schweiger K, et al. Ankle joint pressure in pes cavovarus. J Bone Joint Surg Br 2007;89:1660–5.
48. Beals TC, Manoli A. Late varus instability with equinus deformity. Foot Ankle Surg 1998;4:77–81.
49. Irwin TA, Anderson RB, Davis WH, et al. Effect of ankle arthritis on clinical outcome of lateral ankle ligament reconstruction in cavovarus feet. Foot Ankle Int 2010;31:941–8.
50. Takakura Y, Tanaka Y, Kumai T, et al. Low tibial osteotomy for osteoarthritis of the ankle. J Bone Joint Surg Br 1995;77:50–4.
51. Tanaka Y, Takakura Y, Hayashi K, et al. Low tibial osteotomy for varus-type osteoarthritis of the ankle. J Bone Joint Surg Br 2006;88:909–13.
52. Knupp M, Stufkens SA, Bolliger L, et al. Classification and treatment of supramalleolar deformities. Foot Ankle Int 2011;32:1023–31.

Joint-Sparing Correction for Idiopathic Cavus Foot
Correlation of Clinical and Radiographic Results

Hong-Geun Jung, MD, PhD[a],*, Jong-Tae Park, MD[b],
Sang-Hun Lee, MD[a]

KEYWORDS

- Cavovarus foot • Idiopathic • Joint preservation surgery
- Lateral sliding calcaneal osteotomy • First metatarsal dorsiflexion osteotomy

KEY POINTS

- Difference between idiopathic cavus foot (ICF) and neuromuscular cavus foot (NCF).
- Spectrum of joint preservation surgeries.
- Radiographic parameters for cavovarus foot reconstruction.
- Correlation of clinical and radiographic outcomes of ICF reconstruction.

INTRODUCTION

Pes cavovarus is a complex deformity resulting from plantar flexion of the medial fore-foot, hindfoot varus, and contracture of the plantar soft tissues. Ankle instability is not uncommonly combined. Cavovarus foot deformity often results from muscular imbalance.[1] This imbalance can be of neuromuscular, traumatic, congenital, or idiopathic origin. Relative weakness of the peroneus brevis and tibialis anterior muscles with strong tibialis posterior and peroneus longus muscles cause plantar flexion of the 1st metatarsal bone and varus of the hindfoot. Peripheral neuropathy causes additional weakness of intrinsic foot muscles resulting in a clawfoot deformity.[2]

Neuromuscular cavus foot can be caused by poliomyelitis, cerebrovascular disorder, spinal dysraphism, or hereditary motor sensory neuropathy (HMSN). The cause of ICF is unknown. ICF, however, can be considered a deformity caused by a neurologic disorder not able to be diagnosed specifically.[3] Although an accurate neurologic

[a] Department of Orthopedic Surgery, Konkuk University School of Medicine, 120-1 Neungdong-ro, Hwayang-dong, Gwangjin-gu, Seoul 143-729, South Korea; [b] Department of Orthopedic Surgery, Good Samsun Hospital, 326 Gaya-daero, Sasang-gu, Busan 617-718, South Korea
* Corresponding author.
E-mail address: jungfoot@hanmail.net

Foot Ankle Clin N Am 18 (2013) 659–671
http://dx.doi.org/10.1016/j.fcl.2013.08.003
1083-7515/13/$ – see front matter © 2013 Elsevier Inc. All rights reserved.

(clinical and electrophysiologic) evaluation can identify the cause of cavus foot deformity in some patients, Lelievere asserted that ICF is caused by a neurologic disorder in which the only symptoms are in the cavus foot. Although the degree of deformity overall seems less severe compared with the NCF, the ICF is also a complex deformity with similar features of NCF deformity (ie, a dorsiflexed and varus hindfoot, plantar flexed forefoot, and subsequent elevation of the plantar arch) (**Fig. 1**).[4]

Although cavovarus deformity in children is usually flexible and can be treated with soft tissue procedures, the deformity becomes fixed with time. Adult patients present with rigid cavovarus deformity, where the correction can no longer be obtained using soft tissue procedures alone, and corrective arthrodesis or osteotomy must be performed to realign the deformity. Reconstructive surgeries for cavovarus foot deformities are variable because they include hindfoot or midfoot osteotomy or arthrodesis, soft tissue release or lengthening, tendon transfers, and so forth. Comprehensive evaluation of the spectrum and degree of the deformity and its cause is mandatory to achieve successful deformity correction. This review discusses the patterns of joint-preserving surgical procedures for reconstruction of the ICF and reviews clinical outcomes and their correlations with radiographic outcomes.

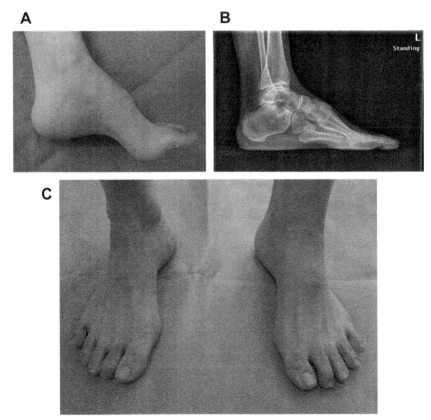

Fig. 1. (*A*) ICF with dorsiflexed and varus hindfoot, plantar flexed forefoot, and subsequent elevation of the plantar arch. (*B*) Simple standing radiograph of the same cavus foot. (*C*) Standing gross view showing high arch and heel varus.

SURGICAL OPTIONS

The surgical options to address idiopathic cavovarus deformity are not significantly different from those used to correct neuromuscular pes cavovarus, although the degree of the deformity is commonly found more pronounced in the NCF compared with the ICF. Because ICF deformity usually does not involve significant muscular imbalance, the posterior tibial tendon or long flexor tendon transfer to foot dorsum to assist ankle dorsiflexion is usually not required.

The surgical procedures are combinations of bony reconstructions and soft tissue procedures. As for the joint-sparing corrective osteotomies, calcaneal osteotomy, 1st metatarsal base dorsiflexion osteotomy (1MTDFO), and midfoot dorsal closing wedge osteotomy at cuneiform-navicular and cuboid level are considered. As for the soft tissue procedures, mainly plantar fascia release, Achilles tendon lengthening, and peroneus longus to brevis tenodesis are most frequent surgical procedures performed. In cases of severe rigid cavus deformities that cannot be addressed with joint-sparing osteotomies, however, triple arthrodesis must be considered, which is beyond of the scope of this article.

Lateral Sliding Calcaneal Osteotomy

Several extra-articular osteotomies have been described to correct the fixed cavovarus foot. These rely on correction through the calcaneus for the hindfoot cavus and varus deformities, whereas the metatarsal or midfoot closing wedge osteotomies are performed to correct the midfoot or forefoot cavus deformities. Dwyer believed the first step in the operative correction of the cavovarus foot was to correct heel varus.[5–7] He reported a good or excellent outcome in 109 of 170 feet that underwent a lateral closing wedge osteotomy of the heel for cavovarus deformity. Although hindfoot varus is compensatory to forefoot cavus and flexible initially, it becomes more rigid with resultant loss of flexibility. The lack of flexibilty ultimately results in a symptomatic cavus foot that prompts the patient to be seen in a clinic.

Therefore, corrective calcaneal osteotomy is almost routinely performed to address the hindfoot varus. This procedure can be accomplished also by lateral closing wedge or biplanar osteotomy (ie, lateral sliding and lateral closing-wedge) or triplanar osteotomy (ie, biplanar with proximal sliding of calcaneal tuberosity to concomitantly decrease the calcaneal pitch angle [CPA]) (**Fig. 2**). Lateral sliding calcaneal osteotomy (LSCO) is mainly performed in oblique fashion, but angular osteotomy or Z-type osteotomy can also be performed. Sammarco and Taylor[8] reported combined metatarsal and calcaneal osteotomies for the treatment of the painful, rigid cavovarus foot in 21 feet; 89% good to excellent outcome was obtained with average follow-up of 49.8 months. Ankle and subtalar range of motion was unchanged or improved in 16 of the 19 feet (84%). The authors usually perform simply LSCO for mild to moderate hindfoot varus deformity, whereas biplanar osteotomy is performed for severe hindfoot varus deformity. Triplanar osteotomy is mostly performed for hindfoot cavovarus deformity. As for the degree of lateral sliding of the calcaneus, approximately 5 mm to 10 mm, 10 mm, and 10 mm to 15 mm lateral translations are performed for mild, moderate, and severe varus deformity, respectively. The authors define mild, moderate, and severe degree of hindfoot varus by tibiocalcaneal axis angle (TCA) of below 10°, 10° to 20°, and above 20°, respectively, measured from hindfoot alignment view. The authors usually resect 5-mm wedge for lateral closing wedge osteotomy to achieve neutral alignment and confirm intraoperatively with image intensifier.

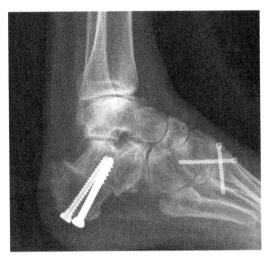

Fig. 2. Triplanar calcaneal osteotomy to concomitantly translate the heel axis laterally, valgization of heel varus, and proximal migration of the distal calcaneal tuberosity to decrease the calcaneal axis.

First Metatarsal Base Dorsiflexion Osteotomy

Osteotomizing 1 or more metatarsals to correct the cavovarus foot deformity was first described by Swanson and colleagues.[9] Gould[10] combined Dwyer's closing wedge calcaneal osteotomy with osteotomies of the proximal metatarsals in 10 of 18 cavovarus feet secondary to Charcot-Marie-Tooth (CMT) disease. Sammarco reported that 21 feet in 15 patients underwent osteotomies of the calcaneus and 1 or more metatarsals for symptomatic cavovarus foot deformity. Complications included nonunion of 3 metatarsal osteotomies and delayed union of 2. The metatarsal nonunions healed after bone grafting; 1 of the 2 delayed unions healed after fixation with a compression screw and 1 healed spontaneously 7 months postoperatively.[8]

1MTDFO is performed to decrease the medial forefoot plantar flexion deformity, where the 1st ray is the main contributor. Oblique osteotomy is started approximately 2 cm to 3 cm distal to the tarsometatarsal (TMT) joint at the dorsum of the metatarsal cortex and directed proximal-plantar approximately 30° caudally, ending proximal to the TMT joint. Dorsal wedge with thickness of 2 mm to 5 mm is removed and fixed with screw after closing the gap by dorsiflexing the distal metatarsal fragment. For severe 1st ray plantar flexion deformity (ie, forefoot cavus), instead of 1MTDFO, 1st TMT dorsiflexion arthrodesis (1TMTDFA) has been performed, which showed higher degree of forefoot cavus correctability compared with 1MTDFO. Although 1TMTDFA sacrifices the 1st TMT joint, the TMT joint originally has a limited motion, especially in cavus foot, and, therefore, does not lead to much loss of joint motion and, therefore, must be differentiated from other major joint fusion surgeries, such as triple arthrodesis (**Fig. 3**). The 1MTDFO is usually performed for mild forefoot cavus versus the 1TMTDFA for moderate and severe forefoot cavus deformity, decided clinically as well as radiographically. In the authors' practice, mostly the 1TMTDFA has been performed for recent cases due to more powerful correctability.

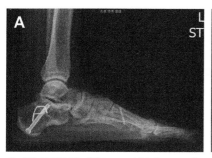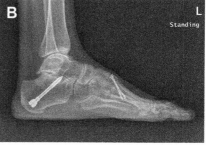

Fig. 3. (A) 1MTDFO. (B) Lateral biplanar calcaneal osteotomy and 1TMTDFA were performed to correct the cavovarus deformity.

Midfoot Dorsal Wedge Osteotomy

Cavus foot can be classified regionally as forefoot, midfoot, and hindfoot cavus. In adult patients who have a fixed cavus foot with its apex at the tarsus (ie, midfoot cavus), dorsal closing wedge osteotomy (DCWO) has been used.[11–13] Wülker and Hurschler[11] reported DCWO for cavus foot deformity in 13 feet with 46 months' follow-up. The dorsally based bone wedge was sized according to the talo-1st metatarsal angle on preoperative radiograph and excised between the Lisfranc and Chopart joint line. In patients with concomitant forefoot adduction, the base of the wedge was excised in a dorsolateral direction but the plantar fascia was left intact. One-third of the patients in their study were not satisfied with the outcome because of the mild to moderate pain, although the patients significantly improved from their preoperative conditions. Strictly speaking, DCWO is not joint preservation surgery and disrupts the naviculocuneiform joint. This violation of the naviculocuneiform joint may play a role in the residual pain patients experience despite the satisfactory postoperative radiographic appearance. Midfoot DCWO, however, can still be an ideal surgical option for severe midfoot cavus foot with apex at the midfoot.

Giannini and colleagues[4] reported 69 feet in 39 patients of ICF treated with plantar fasciotomy, naviculocuneiform arthrodesis, and cuboid osteotomy. There were 2 nonunions at the site of naviculocuneiform arthrodesis and one of them was painful. The mean postoperative Maryland Foot Score was 88%, and 72% of the patients showed good/excellent results. The total ankle range of motion was symmetric, but the mean heel alignment improved from 6° of varus preoperatively to 2° valgus postoperatively. The midfoot DCWO procedure, in contrast with triple arthrodesis, permits correction of a severe midfoot cavus deformity without compromising the tarsal inversion/eversion and dorsoplantar motion of the foot, so that alternating pronation and supination remains possible during gait, reducing the overload of the foot and ankle joints.

Soft Tissue Procedures

Soft tissue release alone, which is indicated in flexible deformities, particularly in children, is no longer applicable in fixed deformities in adults.[11] Once fixed deformity is established in cavovarus foot, correction can no longer be obtained using soft tissue procedures alone and corrective arthrodesis or osteotomy must be used.[14] Soft tissue procedures are performed as adjunctive procedures. Plantar fascia release is commonly performed as an adjunctive procedure to release the contracted plantar fascia, which contributes to the high medial longitudinal arch.

Lateral ligament reconstruction should be concomitantly performed in cases of combined chronic lateral ankle instability. The major ligament reconstruction procedures commonly performed are the modified Chrisman-Snook procedure and peroneus longus to brevis transfer. In order for these ligament reconstruction procedures to be effective and long lasting, the hindfoot varus deformity should be realigned by bony correction before the ligament reconstruction. The modified Chrisman-Snook procedure is a powerful static ligament stabilizer utilizing the anterior half of the peroneus brevis tendon, whereas the peroneus longus to brevis transfer procedure is a dynamic stabilizer of the lateral ankle that removes the 1st ray plantar flexion power by peroneus longus, which contributes to forefoot cavus deformity and augments the lateral ankle stabilizing power by tenodesing to the peroneus brevis tendon. In cases of clinically severe lateral ankle instability, however, the modified Chrisman-Snook procedure is more effective in stabilizing the unstable lateral ankle, although it is more invasive surgically. In the authors' practice, the modified Chrisman-Snook procedure and peroneus longus to brevis transfer have not been performed concomitantly. The modified Chrisman-Snook procedure is indicated for moderate to severe lateral ankle instability whereas the peroneus longus to brevis transfer is for mild or subtle instability patients.

CLINICAL AND RADIOGRAPHIC OUTCOME CORRELATION

As for the radiographic parameters to measure the degree of cavus deformity correction radiographically, the CPA, Meary angle (lateral talo-1st metatarsal angle [LT1MTA]), arch angle (AA), and navicular height are measured in standing foot lateral radiograph and the TCA is measured at the hindfoot alignment view radiograph (**Fig. 4**).

Kroon and colleagues[15] reported the clinical outcome of joint preservation surgery for correction of flexible pes cavovarus in 15 adults. Their results showed that in joint-preserving flexible pes cavovarus correction, patient satisfaction was generally good. Radiographic alignment of the foot was not significantly associated with patient-based outcome. The anatomic corrections of the foot (preoperative and postoperative TMT I angle and CPA as well as the change in TMT I angle and CPA) did not show any association with the clinical characteristics of the patients (foot function index [FFI], American Orthopaedic Foot and Ankle Society [AOFAS] score, alignment, ankle range of motion, and patient satisfaction).[15] The success of the treatment is highly dependent on individualization of the procedure.[16] Radiographic analysis revealed a decrease in forefoot adduction (average 9.6°) and a reduction in both hindfoot (average 9.1°) and forefoot cavus (10.6°), leading to an overall 13% reduction in the height of the longitudinal arch. All changes were statistically significant (*P*<.05).[8]

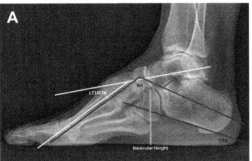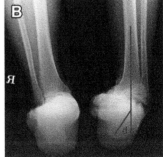

Fig. 4. (*A*) CPA, Meary angle (LT1MTA), AA, and navicular height. (*B*) TCA is measured in hindfoot alignment view.

The authors' current study of ICF reconstruction (9 feet), mainly calcaneal and metatarsal osteotomies, showed that ankle hindfoot AOFAS score improved from 56.8 (42–75) to 89.2 (66–100) postoperatively ($P = .008$) and the visual analog scale (VAS) score improved form 3.8 (0–9) to 1.3 (0–5) postoperatively ($P<.05$) The CPA in the authors' current study decreased from average 21.3° to 18.6° postoperatively ($P>.05$); however, radiographic measures, such as Meary angle, improved from 15.2° to 7.6°, AA decreased from 49.5° to 40.6°, navicular height decreased from 52.2 mm to 41.0 mm, and TCA markedly decreased from varus 7.1° to valgus 1.0° postoperatively, all with statistical significance (**Table 1**). Generally, although the osteotomies were performed to create significant correction of the deformity and clinically the patients showed marked functional improvement, the radiographic results overall did not show significant change postoperatively. Among the radiographic measurements, the TCA angle measured from hindfoot alignment view showed most significant degree of improvement after bony reconstruction for the cavovarus foot deformity (**Fig. 5**). The authors' results showed that although the degree of normal foot realignment, measured on radiographs, is the ultimate goal of the surgical correction leading to plantigrade foot and improves patient function postoperatively, it does not significantly correlate with the degree of pain relief or functional improvement ($P>.05$). This finding is in agreement with previous studies in surgical clubfoot correction.[17,18] A possible explanation for satisfactory results is that the restored muscle balance due to reconstruction is the most important feature. If balance cannot be restored due to lack of muscle function, triple arthrodesis or ankle fusion should be performed. Triple arthrodesis has more frequent occurrence of pseudoarthrosis, however, in particular the talonavicular joint and degenerative changes of the adjacent joints in the long term.[19]

Ward and colleagues[20] treated patients with CMT disease and flexible cavovarus foot deformity with a reconstruction consisting mainly of dorsiflexion osteotomy of the 1st metatarsal, transfer of the peroneus longus to the peroneus brevis, and plantar fascia release without calacaneal osteotomy. Radiographic analysis revealed that some hindfoot varus recurred in most patients. The authors attributed the cause of the hindfoot varus recurrence to the soleus muscle inversion power. The authors, however, think that the adult flexible cavovarus feet still possess variable degree of rigidity in the varus hindfoot, although the major cause is compensatory of the 1st metatarsal plantar flexion, and that calcaneal osteotomy, whether it is simply lateral sliding or biplanar or triplanar osteotomy, is required in almost all cases to adequately address the hindfoot varus deformity. After bony reconstruction (ie, mainly calcaneal osteotomy and 1MTDFO or 1TMTDFA and additional soft tissue reconstruction), most patients experienced marked clinical improvement in the aspect of weight bearing, ambulation, and so forth. The authors also found significant change or improvement of most of the radiographic parameters related to the cavovarus deformity after reconstruction, except the CPA.

Adult patients with cavovarus feet were seen with symptomatic ankle arthrosis and frequently lateral hindfoot instability. Once a fixed cavovarus deformity occurs, it can alter biomechanical contact stress and contact area leading to thin articular cartilage and arthritis (**Fig. 6**).[21] Cavovarus foot realignment with anteromedial ankle chilectomy reliably improved patients' symptoms related to ankle arthrosis and stabilized the extent of anteromedial ankle arthrosis when talar varus tilt was reduced.[22]

DISCUSSION

In cavovarus foot, the muscle involvement progresses from distal to proximal, affecting primarily the tibialis anterior and peroneus brevis, with secondary

Table 1
Joint preservation surgeries for the cavovarus foot deformities

Author, Year	No.	Follow-up (mo)	Etiology	Main Surgical Procedures	Clinical Outcome	Patient Satisfaction	Radiographic Outcome		
							CPA	LT1MTA	TCA
Sammarco & Taylor,[8] 2001	21	49.8	HMSN, postpolio, etc.	Lateral sliding calcaneal osteotomy, dorsolateral closing wedge osteotomy of metatarsal base(s)	AOFAS score 40.9→89.1 Maryland Foot Score 72.1→89.9	—	Average correction −9.1°	Average correction −6.5°	—
Wülker & Hurschler,[11] 2002	13	46	—	Midfoot DCWO	—	Satisfied (9)	—	Mean 14° Average correction 23°	—
Giannini et al,[4] 2002	69	84	Idiopathic	Naviculocuneiform joint resection arthrodesis, cuboid closing wedge osteotomy, open plantar fasciotomy,	Maryland Foot Score postoperative 88	Excellent (33%), good (39%), fair (25%), poor (3%)	—	—	—

Study	No.		Diagnosis	Procedure	Outcome	Satisfaction			
Kroon et al,[15] 2010	19	50	HMSN, encephalopathy, spina bifida, idiopathic	Lateral sliding calcaneal osteotomy, 1st MT DCWO, soft tissue releases, tendon transfer and lengthening	AOFAS score postoperative 82.5 ± 16	Very satisfied (5), satisfied (10), moderately (2), unsatisfied (2)	153 ± 6.8° →152 ± 6.7°	23 ± 4.6° →17 ± 4.2°	—
Maskill et al,[31] 2010	29	53	Subtle cavovarus	Lateral sliding calcaneal osteotomy, 1st MT DCWO, peroneus longus to brevis transfer, Achilles tendon lengthening	AOFAS score 45→90	—	26.1°→22.7°	9.9°→2.4°	—
Leeuwesteijn et al,[35] 2010	52	56.9	CMT disease	1st MT DCWO, Achilles tendon lengthening	FFI score for pain 29.3%→14.8% Disability 37.8%→23.5%	Satisfied (90%)	—	—	—

Abbreviations: MT, metatarsal; No., number of feet; →, change of values.

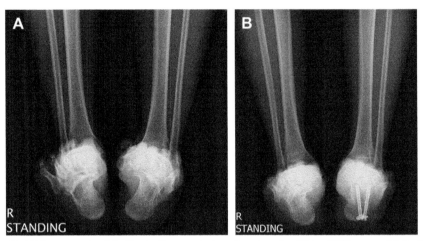

Fig. 5. (A) Preoperative hindfoot alignment view showing the TCA of 20° varus. (B) Postbiplanar calcaneal osteotomy showing 3° varus TCA.

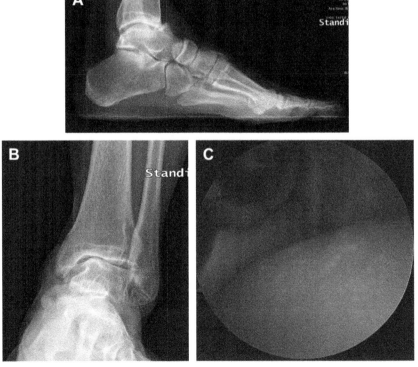

Fig. 6. ICF with ankle osteoarthritis (OA). (A) Preoperative foot lateral. (B) Preoperative ankle anteroposterior showing ankle OA with tilted talus. (C) Denuded ankle cartilage showing advanced OA.

dysfunction of the intrinsic muscles. Relative sparing of extensor hallucis longus is observed. The weakness of the anterior tibialis relative to the peroneus longus results in plantar flexion of the 1st metatarsal. Secondary to weakness of the tibialis, anterior recruitment of extensor hallucis longus occurs, resulting in cock-up deformity of the 1st toe, with further depression of the metatarsal head and plantar contracture.[23] The forefoot cavus deformity forces the hindfoot into varus. The deformity of the hind-foot initially is flexible but can become rigid over time. Decreased strength of the intrinsic muscles results in unopposed action of the extrinsic musculature (extensor digitorum longus and flexor digitorum longus). This increases equinus and results in claw toes.[24]

A wide variety of surgical procedures have been described for the treatment of cavovarus foot deformity and varying degrees of success reported. These procedures include plantar release, calcaneal osteotomy,[25] metatarsal osteotomies,[26] TMT osteotomies, tarsal osteotomy,[27,28] and various tendon transfers. Typically, patients undergo any number of soft-tissue procedures while the deformity is flexible and additional osseous procedures when the deformity becomes rigid. In the 3 studies in which patients were followed for more than 5 years, no single procedure or combination of procedures was found to offer consistently good long-term results[29,30]; 35 consecutive patients with lateral-based symptoms due to an underlying congenital subtle cavovarus foot type were surgically corrected. Various procedures were used, including some combination of the following: lateral displacement calcaneus osteotomy, peroneus longus to brevis transfer, dorsiflexion 1st metatarsal osteotomy, and Achilles tendon lengthening. The mean AOFAS ankle hindfoot score preoperatively was 45 and postoperatively was 90.[31]

In the past, many patients with CMT disease and cavovarus foot deformity have undergone triple arthrodesis, previously considered a definitive procedure to create a well-aligned, functional foot.[29,30] Long-term follow-up studies have shown, however, a high incidence of osteoarthritis of the remaining foot joints after this procedure. Triple arthrodesis has historically been the treatment of choice for the painful, cavovarus foot with fixed deformity. Although triple arthrodesis may restore a plantigrade foot, it does so at the expense of subtalar and transverse tarsal joint motion.[32] Drennan reported symptomatic ankle arthritis in 19 of 30 patients who underwent triple arthrodesis for CMT disease.[33] Other reported complications include neuroarthropathy, pseudarthrosis, residual deformity, midfoot arthritis, and avascular necrosis of the talus.[30]

Tarsal-metatarsal arthrodesis through a dorsal closing wedge to correct cavovarus foot deformity was described by Jahss.[13] Gellman and colleagues[34] demonstrated that 21% of dorsiflexion, 10% of plantarflexion, 12% of inversion, and 16% of eversion in the foot occur through the metatarsal-cuneiform joints. Although arthrodesis of the tarsal-metatarsal joint preserves midfoot and hindfoot motion, the motion and shock-absorbing effect of the metatarsal-cuneiform-cuboid complex is lost.[8]

Therefore, the authors conclude that recently the adult cavovarus foot deformities have been more commonly addressed with joint preservation osteotomies and adjunctive soft tissue surgeries and less with triple arthrodesis. From the reports, clinical and radiographic outcome are overall favorable, although the radiographic changes did not lead to perfect correction. The clinical and radiographic outcomes did not show positive correlation. Surgically, it is difficult to achieve normal radiographic realignment for the cavovarus deformity, although clinically, patients improve significantly the gross forefoot cavus and hindfoot varus deformity as well as showing marked pain and functional improvement. Radiographs do not seem to fully reflect the magnitude of surgical correction. In summary, the LSCO calcaneal osteotomy and the 1MTDFO or 1TMTDFA are 2 most important surgical procedures to address the cavovarus deformities and it must be emphasized that the amount of their corrections need to be adequate enough to achieve neutral heel alignment and 0° LT1MTA and lead to satisfactory clinical results.

REFERENCES

1. Charles YP, Louahem D, Dimeglio A. Cavovarus foot deformity with multiple tarsal coalitions: functional and three-dimensional preoperative assessment. J Foot Ankle Surg 2006;45(2):118.
2. Aminian A, Sangeorzan BJ. The anatomy of cavus foot deformity. Foot Ankle Clin 2008;13(2):191.
3. Brewerton DA, Sandifer PH, Sweetnam DR. "Idiopathic" Pes Cavus: an investigation into its aetiology. Br Med J 1963;2(5358):659.
4. Giannini S, Ceccarelli F, Benedetti MG, et al. Surgical treatment of adult idiopathic cavus foot with plantar fasciotomy, naviculocuneiform arthrodesis, and cuboid osteotomy. A review of thirty-nine cases. J Bone Joint Surg Am 2002; 84(Suppl 2):62.
5. Dwyer FC. Osteotomy of the calcaneum for pes cavus. J Bone Joint Surg Br 1959;41(1):80.
6. Dwyer FC. The present status of the problem of pes cavus. Clin Orthop Relat Res 1975;(106):254.
7. Boffeli TJ, Collier RC. Surgical technique for combined Dwyer calcaneal osteotomy and peroneal tendon repair for correction of peroneal tendon pathology associated with cavus foot deformity. J Foot Ankle Surg 2012;51(1):135.
8. Sammarco GJ, Taylor R. Cavovarus foot treated with combined calcaneus and metatarsal osteotomies. Foot Ankle Int 2001;22(1):19.
9. Swanson AB, Browne HS, Coreman JD. The cavus foot-concepts of production and treatment by metatarsal osteotomy. J Bone Joint Surg Am 1966;48(5): 1019.
10. Gould N. Surgery in advanced Charcot-Marie-Tooth disease. Foot Ankle 1984; 4(5):267.
11. Wülker N, Hurschler C. Cavus foot correction in adults by dorsal closing wedge osteotomy. Foot Ankle Int 2002;23(4):344.
12. Jahss MH. Evaluation of the cavus foot for orthopedic treatment. Clin Orthop Relat Res 1983;(181):52.
13. Jahss MH. Tarsometatarsal truncated-wedge arthrodesis for pes cavus and equinovarus deformity of the fore part of the foot. J Bone Joint Surg Am 1980;62(5): 713.
14. Samilson RL, Dillin W. Cavus, cavovarus, and calcaneocavus. An update. Clin Orthop Relat Res 1983;(177):125.
15. Kroon M, Faber FW, van der Linden M. Joint preservation surgery for correction of flexible pes cavovarus in adults. Foot Ankle Int 2010;31(1):24.
16. Watanabe RS. Metatarsal osteotomy for the cavus foot. Clin Orthop Relat Res 1990;(252):217.
17. Cooper DM, Dietz FR. Treatment of idiopathic clubfoot. A thirty-year follow-up note. J Bone Joint Surg Am 1995;77(10):1477.
18. Herbsthofer B, Eckardt A, Rompe JD, et al. Significance of radiographic angle measurements in evaluation of congenital clubfoot. Arch Orthop Trauma Surg 1998;117(6–7):324.
19. Azmaipairashvili Z, Riddle EC, Scavina M, et al. Correction of cavovarus foot deformity in Charcot-Marie-Tooth disease. J Pediatr Orthop 2005;25(3):360.

20. Ward CM, Dolan LA, Bennett DL, et al. Long-term results of reconstruction for treatment of a flexible cavovarus foot in Charcot-Marie-Tooth disease. J Bone Joint Surg Am 2008;90(12):2631.

21. LaClair SM. Reconstruction of the varus ankle from soft-tissue procedures with osteotomy through arthrodesis. Foot Ankle Clin 2007;12(1):153.

22. Krause FG, Henning J, Pfander G, et al. Cavovarus foot realignment to treat anteromedial ankle arthrosis. Foot Ankle Int 2013;34(1):54.

23. Ortiz C, Wagner E, Keller A. Cavovarus foot reconstruction. Foot Ankle Clin 2009; 14(3):471.

24. Marks RM. Midfoot and forefoot issues cavovarus foot: assessment and treatment issues. Foot Ankle Clin 2008;13(2):229.

25. Mitchell GP. Posterior displacement osteotomy of the calcaneus. J Bone Joint Surg Br 1977;59(2):233.

26. Thomas FB. Levelling the tread. Elevation of the dropped metatarsal head by metatarsal osteotomy. J Bone Joint Surg Br 1974;56(2):314.

27. Wilcox PG, Weiner DS. The Akron midtarsal dome osteotomy in the treatment of rigid pes cavus: a preliminary review. J Pediatr Orthop 1985;5(3):333.

28. Wicart P, Seringe R. Plantar opening-wedge osteotomy of cuneiform bones combined with selective plantar release and dwyer osteotomy for pes cavovarus in children. J Pediatr Orthop 2006;26(1):100.

29. Wukich DK, Bowen JR. A long-term study of triple arthrodesis for correction of pes cavovarus in Charcot-Marie-Tooth disease. J Pediatr Orthop 1989;9(4):433.

30. Mann DC, Hsu JD. Triple arthrodesis in the treatment of fixed cavovarus deformity in adolescent patients with Charcot-Marie-Tooth disease. Foot Ankle 1992;13(1):1.

31. Maskill MP, Maskill JD, Pomeroy GC. Surgical management and treatment algorithm for the subtle cavovarus foot. Foot Ankle Int 2010;31(12):1057.

32. Siffert RS, del Torto U. "Beak" triple arthrodesis for severe cavus deformity. Clin Orthop Relat Res 1983;(181):64.

33. Wetmore RS, Drennan JC. Long-term results of triple arthrodesis in Charcot-Marie-Tooth disease. J Bone Joint Surg Am 1989;71(3):417-22.

34. Gellman H, Lenihan M, Halikis N, et al. Selective tarsal arthrodesis: an in vitro analysis of the effect on foot motion. Foot Ankle 1987;8(3):127-33.

35. Leeuwesteijn AE, de Visser E, Louwerens JW, et al. Flexible cavovarus feet in Charcot-Marie-Tooth disease treated with first ray proximal dorsiflexion osteotomy combined with soft tissue surgery: a short-term to mid-term outcome study. Foot Ankle Surg 2010 Sep;16(3):142-7.

Joint Sparing Correction of Cavovarus Feet in Charcot-Marie-Tooth Disease

What Are the Limits?

Tristan Barton, MBChB, FRCS[a],*, Ian Winson, MBChB, FRCS[b]

KEYWORDS

- Charcot-Marie-Tooth • Cavovarus • Osteotomy • Tendon transfers • Arthrodesis

KEY POINTS

- Foot deformity in the patient with Charcot-Marie-Tooth (CMT) disease frequently presents in the young patient with symptoms such as abnormal gait, forefoot pain, ankle instability, and changing foot posture.
- Due to the poor outcomes associated with both nonoperative management and triple arthrodesis, joint sparing surgery is the preferable treatment option.
- Numerous surgical procedures have been described, all with the aim of achieving a plantigrade and balanced foot.
- The surgery must be tailored to the requirements of the individual patient and involves a combination of soft-tissue releases, tendon transfers, and osteotomies.
- The outcomes reported in the literature are variable but suggest that joint sparing surgery in young patients with CMT disease is a viable and a preferable alternative to triple arthrodesis.

INTRODUCTION

CMT disease was described independently in 1886 by Jean-Martin Charcot and his pupil Pierre Marie in France, and Howard Henry Tooth in England.[1,2] CMT disease is the most common inherited neuropathy, with an incidence of 1 in 2500 in the United States of America.[3] With advances in genetic testing, it is now understood that this condition is a group of diseases, resulting from defects in the genetic code for the protein of the peripheral myelin sheath. More than 30 genetic defects have now been identified, with the most common form being CMT disease type 1A. This

[a] Department of Trauma and Orthopaedics, Royal United Hospital Bath NHS Trust, Combe Park, Bath, BA1 3NG, UK; [b] Department of Trauma and Orthopaedics, Avon Orthopaedic Centre, Southmead Hospital, Westbury-on-Trym, Bristol BS10 5NB, UK
* Corresponding author.
E-mail address: tristan_barton@hotmail.com

Foot Ankle Clin N Am 18 (2013) 673–688
http://dx.doi.org/10.1016/j.fcl.2013.08.008
1083-7515/13/$ – see front matter Crown Copyright © 2013 Published by Elsevier Inc. All rights reserved.

variation of the disease is the consequence of a defect on chromosome 17 coding for peripheral myelin protein 22, which causes a reduction in peripheral nerve conduction velocities and resultant distal muscle weakness. In type 2 CMT disease, the pathophysiology of muscle weakness is different. There is no evidence of axonal demyelination, and there is a reduced amplitude rather than velocity of the nerve impulses.

The pattern of distal muscle weakness in CMT disease is unusual in that it is selective. Within a lower limb myofascial compartment, individual muscle weakness is variable in both the timing of its onset and the severity of the involvement. It is this imbalance in muscle involvement that causes the resultant foot deformities characteristically seen in CMT disease. This imbalance becomes more apparent as a child grows, and therefore children most often present with lower limb symptoms during periods of accelerated growth such as adolescence.

In treating foot deformities in patients with CMT disease, the orthopedic surgeon needs to recognize several key issues. First, the pattern of muscle involvement is not consistent, and this variation in genotype expression is best illustrated in families with CMT disease. Family members with identical genotypes can display marked phenotypic variation. Each patient must be examined to assess precisely the involvement of each individual muscle, which is of paramount importance if the deformity is to be understood and correctly treated. It is of course true that other genetically determined characteristics of the foot are completely separate to this, for example, that hypermobility or bone length can influence how the genotype is expressed.

Second, the disease process is progressive rather than static. If the muscle imbalances are not addressed, the deformities worsen. There is little in the literature to guide the surgeon as to when to intervene, and evidence is principally anecdotal. The consensus among surgeons is that there is little role for nonsurgical management of the progressive foot deformity in patients with CMT disease. If left untreated, the deformity worsens due to both disease progression and persisting muscle imbalances.

Third, patients frequently present at a young age. In the older patient with a long-standing fixed foot deformity and associated degenerative changes, the decision-making process is simplified. Such patients require joint sacrificing surgery with additional muscle balancing as required.[4] In the young patient, the aim must be to preserve joint motion, balance the foot, and prevent the progression to a fixed and symptomatic deformity.

Nonoperative treatment of the progressive foot deformity in patients with CMT disease is recognized as producing unsatisfactory results.[5] Surgical options for the treatment of CMT disease are joint preserving, joint sacrificing, or a combination of these 2 approaches. Although there is little evidence in the literature directly comparing the various surgical options, the recent trend is toward joint preserving surgery in young patients. The basis for this shift is the poor long-term results of patients who have undergone a triple arthrodesis in childhood for a foot deformity secondary to CMT disease. At the very least, by sacrificing the joints early, the number of surgical options available at a later date is reduced. Just possibly by changing the deforming forces and balancing the foot, later destructive changes are prevented.

Wukich and Bowen[6] reported that of 22 patients reviewed after triple arthrodesis at 12 years, only 32% had a good objective result. About 88% of patients, however, reported good to excellent function, and 86% were satisfied. Wetmore and Drennan[7] reported less satisfactory results after 30 triple arthrodeses in 16 patients. They found only 24% of patients reported good or excellent results, compared with 77% reporting fair or poor results. A total of 23 patients developed degenerative changes in the surrounding joints, with 6 patients requiring an ankle arthrodesis. Seven patients had a recurrence of the deformity. Mann and Hsu[8] reported on the 7-year results after triple arthrodesis. They reported 8 of 12 feet to be asymptomatic; 3 feet were symptomatic secondary to a nonplantigrade foot, and 1 patient required revision.

Triple arthrodesis for static cavovarus deformities such as those secondary to poliomyelitis have more reliable results when compared with the progressive deformity in patients with CMT disease. Despite this, there are patients with CMT disease presenting with degenerative changes in the hindfoot in whom the only reliable surgical option is a triple arthrodesis.

Joint preserving surgery most commonly is performed as a combination of both bony and soft-tissue procedures. The exact nature of the surgery performed must be individualized to correcting the deformities present and neutralizing the forces that produce them.

MOTOR IMBALANCE IN CHARCOT-MARIE-TOOTH DISEASE

The presenting lower limb symptoms in patients with CMT disease can be directly attributed to the muscle imbalance of the foot and ankle complex. Muscle weakness is selective, but the deformities that develop are predictable. Muscle strength testing and magnetic resonance imaging (MRI) studies have confirmed that within a lower leg compartment, muscle involvement is not uniform. In the lateral compartment, peroneus longus function remains preserved, in contrast to the weakness and atrophy demonstrated in the peroneus brevis muscle.[9,10] In the anterior compartment, similar findings are seen with a weak tibialis anterior muscle contrasting with the often-preserved function of extensor hallucis longus (EHL). The posterior compartment muscle function seems to be preserved until later in the disease process, in stark contrast to the intrinsic muscles of the foot that are frequently the first muscles to be affected. CMT disease affects all muscles of the lower limb, but at different stages of the disease process and with varying degrees of severity. The resultant deformities are a consequence of the muscle imbalance between agonists and antagonists.

Weakness of the intrinsic muscles of the foot leads to the typical claw toe deformities of the cavus foot. As a consequence of intrinsic weakness, the unopposed action of the long extensors across the metatarsophalangeal (MTP) joints leads to hyperextension at these joints. The continued action of the long toe flexors (flexor digitorum longus) results in flexion of the interphalangeal (IP) joints and the clawing deformities. These deformities are initially mobile and correctable. An additional effect of the lesser toe deformities is on the medial longitudinal arch. Dorsal subluxation of the phalanges at the MTP joints results in a distal shift of the plantar plate and its attachments to the fat pad. This distal migration and increased dorsiflexion of the toe position means that the plantar fascia is now under increased tension by the windlass mechanism.

MRI studies have demonstrated that a cavus deformity of the foot can result from intrinsic muscle loss in the presence of a preserved Peroneus Longus.[11] In the CMT deformity, peroneus longus is stronger than peroneus brevis and the weak tibialis anterior muscle. As a consequence, with the first metatarsal fixed to the floor during stance, peroneus longus contraction results in the cuboid being pushed under the navicular. This deformity fixes the height of the longitudinal arch resulting in the forefoot being pronated and the hindfoot inverting via a supple subtalar joint. The advanced plantar fascia and the inverting action of tibialis posterior further accentuate this. Peroneus brevis weakness means it is unable to provide a sufficient eversion force to counteract this.

A final functional component to the deformity is a weakness in dorsiflexion as a consequence of a weak tibialis anterior. The degree of tibialis anterior involvement is variable but, if weak, is overpowered by the stronger plantar flexors of the preserved posterior compartment. If the plantar flexion forces are allowed to dominate, then an equinus deformity develops, which prevents passive reduction of the hindfoot varus. To retain active ankle dorsiflexion during gait, the long extensors of the toes are recruited to provide adequate foot clearance, and this in turn worsens the claw toe deformities. This condition is most accentuated in the hallux. Preservation of EHL results in its recruitment as an ankle dorsiflexor. This overactivity combined with weakened foot intrinsics results in marked clawing of the hallux, with the easily recognizable hyperextension of the MTP joint and hyperflexion of the IP joint (due to preservation of flexor hallucis longus within the posterior compartment).

Initially, all the described deformities are flexible and reversible. The longer the muscle imbalance remains the stiffer and less adaptable the foot becomes. Surgery performed on a flexible foot can increase the likelihood of joint preservation and also arrest further deterioration of the deformities by balancing of the affected muscles. The pattern of muscle weakness is variable, and careful assessment is required to evaluate which deformities to correct and which tendon transfers are most appropriate to prevent recurrence.

PATIENT EVALUATION AS A GUIDE TO SURGICAL MANAGEMENT

Patients rarely present before teenage years, although subtle preceding signs and symptoms may have been evident. A careful history may reveal symptoms of early muscle fatigability, a high-stepping gait due to weak ankle dorsiflexors and associated unsteadiness. As the child gets older, the symptoms begin to interfere more with activities of daily living. They may complain of forefoot pain and callosities beneath the first and fifth metatarsal heads and difficulty in obtaining shoe wear due to developing deformities. With the development of a varus hindfoot deformity, the patient may present with recurrent episodes of ankle instability and a previously undiagnosed underlying foot deformity. The surgical approach to addressing the cavovarus foot must be on an individualized basis, and the most critical component of evaluating the foot deformity in a patient with CMT for surgery is the clinical examination. Further imaging is certainly a useful adjunct, but the exact nature of the surgery required is based on the physical examination.

JOINT SPARING SURGICAL OPTIONS

Gould[12] stated that the aim of surgery in the cavovarus foot in patients with CMT disease is to achieve a foot that is

- Plantigrade
- Mobile
- Pain free

The literature describes a multitude of surgical options to achieve these aims, each with its own merits and disadvantages. If a balanced, mobile, and asymptomatic foot is achieved after surgery, then the operative intervention is considered a success. Thought must be given to the presence of degenerative changes, the overall foot alignment, and the muscle imbalances causing the deformities. There is no standard surgical plan for these patients, and each requires an individualized series of procedures to successfully address each of the aforementioned conditions.

HINDFOOT SURGERY

The degree of involvement of each joint must be assessed and deformities evaluated as to whether they are fixed, partially correctable, or fully correctable. Longstanding malalignment leads to secondary degenerative changes in the hindfoot joints, and this must be recognized, as well as how symptomatic these changes are to the patient. The decision as to whether to attempt joint preserving surgery becomes more complicated in the young patient with symptomatic degenerative changes. If degenerative changes are apparent and the joints painful, then the question is how tolerant the affected joints are to such changes. In addition, an understanding is required as to whether realignment surgery would result in deterioration or improvement in the patients' symptoms.

Maintaining ankle motion is a priority when planning hindfoot surgery, and the ankle seems most tolerant of degenerative changes. If less than one-third of the ankle joint is affected (most frequently the anteromedial portion of the ankle joint in the cavovarus deformity) (**Fig. 1**), then realignment redistributes the forces across the joint and allows a mobile joint relatively free of symptoms.[13] If greater than one-third of the ankle joint has degenerative changes evident, then the results are less predictable. In such patients, realignment surgery of the foot remains a necessity to correct and prevent progression of the deformity, as well as normalize pressures across the ankle joint and slow the progression of any degenerative changes. However, symptomatic relief from the ankle itself is unreliable. Such patients must be aware of this possibility before surgery, so expectations remain realistic. Preserving ankle motion in young patients slows the onset of degenerative changes elsewhere

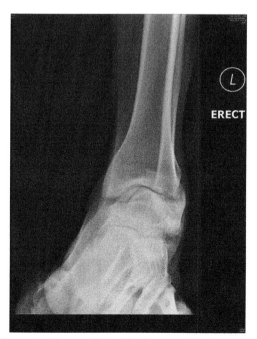

Fig. 1. Radiograph demonstrating medial ankle degenerative changes secondary to a varus hindfoot deformity.

in the foot and ankle complex. To maintain such movement, a degree of pain and stiffness from the ankle may have to be tolerated.

The subtalar and talonavicular joints are less forgiving, and degenerative changes in these joints often remain sufficiently symptomatic. As discussed previously, triple arthrodesis in young patients has less predictable and often less-than-satisfactory results in the longer term. It therefore remains a difficult decision as to when to proceed to such joint sacrificing surgery in these joints. A thorough assessment combined with appropriate imaging of the subtalar joint in particular must be performed to attain the exact source of hindfoot pain. It is preferable to proceed with joint sparing surgery if possible, again in a well-counseled patient who is aware of the possibility of further surgery should symptoms persist.

Hindfoot Alignment

The varus position of the hindfoot must be assessed using any of the described techniques; the most commonly used being the Coleman block test.[14] Other researchers have described tests of hindfoot flexibility in the kneeling or prone position, but the basis of the examination remains the same.[15,16] The key is to first ascertain whether the hindfoot varus is fixed or flexible.

The Coleman Block Test

This test requires the patient to stand fully weight bearing on a block, with the heel and the lateral border of the foot on the block and the first, second, and third metatarsal heads allowed to hang unsupported (Coleman) (**Figs. 2** and **3**). This position allows the medial metatarsals to plantar flex and the forefoot to pronate. The block is approximately 2.5 cm thick and must be appropriate to the size of the patient's foot being assessed. If the hindfoot varus remains (when examined from the back of the patient), then the deformity is fixed. However, if the hindfoot corrects to physiologic valgus (5°), then the deformity is flexible and driven by the forefoot deformity. In reality, the hindfoot varus frequently partially corrects, and in these instances, it is important to see whether the heel corrects beyond neutral (0°) or remains either in neutral or a varus position.

In patients with CMT disease, this test remains a vital tool in assessing the need for corrective hindfoot surgery. If the hindfoot varus is flexible and forefoot driven, the correction of the forefoot deformity results in hindfoot realignment. In such instances, a valgising calcaneal osteotomy is not required. If the hindfoot varus is fixed, then such an osteotomy is required to correct the hindfoot deformity.

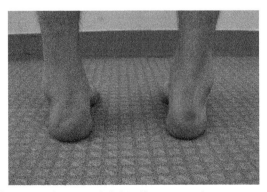

Fig. 2. Right hindfoot varus (previous left hindfoot surgery).

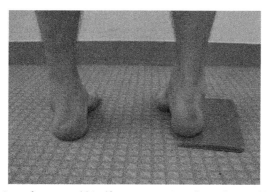

Fig. 3. Demonstration of corrected hindfoot varus using the Coleman block technique.

The hindfoot deformity is frequently partially correctable when assessed using the Coleman block technique. The key to managing hindfoot alignment in such patients is to err on overcorrection rather than on undercorrection; this is due to patients tolerating a varus hindfoot poorly. If the hindfoot is not fully correctable to a valgus position and remains in a varus or even neutral position, then a valgising calcaneal osteotomy should be considered.

Calcaneal Osteotomies

There are numerous techniques for achieving such a hindfoot correction, each with its merits. The simplest osteotomy of the os calcis is a biplanar oblique osteotomy. This single osteotomy allows varying degrees of correction by sliding the tuberosity in both the sagittal and coronal planes. By mobilizing the tuberosity in both a lateral and a cephalad direction, both the varus deformity and the increased calcaneal pitch seen in the cavus foot can be corrected. In addition, the calcaneal length should be increased or decreased by adjusting the angle of the osteotomy in the axial plane. Intrinsic to being able to maintain the osteotomy in the corrected position are modern fixation techniques.

In the more severe varus deformities, a Dwyer osteotomy allows a greater correction in the coronal plane using a laterally based closing wedge osteotomy.[17] The difficulty is, however, that it tends to decrease the length of the calcaneum, and shoe fitting is more difficult. Multiplanar osteotomies such as the crescenteric and 'Z' osteotomies are more complex to perform but allow the surgeon greater flexibility.[18,19] The 'Z' osteotomy combines a lateral translation of the os calcis with a rotation in the axial plane to maximize the potential correction in a stable configuration. The addition of a closing wedge osteotomy increases the corrective power of such an osteotomy without creating any secondary shortening as would occur following a Dwyer.

The senior author's (IGW) preference is to perform a biplanar oblique osteotomy cut across the calcaneum from lateral to medial just in front of the tuberosity and the weight-bearing area, stabilized with a single 6.5-mm cannulated screw into the anterior process (**Fig. 6**). Nonunion or redisplacement have not been seen with this technique.

Forefoot and Midfoot Osteotomies

The position of joints that are passively correctable are corrected by soft-tissue balancing. In the cavovarus foot, the forefoot pronation deformity becomes fixed at an early stage, before any loss of hindfoot mobility. Hindfoot varus often remains correctable until a later stage in the disease process. Once the forefoot deformity becomes fixed, osteotomies are required to re-create a plantigrade foot.

Dorsiflexion osteotomy of the first metatarsal

If the first ray is fixed relative to mobile lesser metatarsals (metatarsals 2–5), then a basal dorsiflexion osteotomy of the first metatarsal is indicated[12,20–26]; this elevates the first metatarsal head and corrects the forefoot pronation when weight bearing. In the authors' institution, such a procedure is carried out via a proximal dorsal closing wedge osteotomy of the first metatarsal. The plantar cortex is preserved to enhance the stability of the osteotomy, which is fixed with either a staple or a 2-hole plate. Depending on other surgeries performed, a patient may start to weight bear through such an osteotomy.

Dorsiflexion midfoot osteotomies

If there is a fixed plantaris deformity across the midfoot, then a more extensive osteotomy is required (**Figs. 4** and **5**). In this situation, there is a fixed pronation and plantaris deformity of the midfoot that involves all the metatarsals, with the apex of the deformity at the level of the cuneiforms and cuboid. A dorsiflexion osteotomy of the first ray is not sufficient in such patients because of the fixed relationship between the first and the lateral metatarsals and a more extensive osteotomy across the midfoot is required. This procedure is performed using multiple dorsal metatarsal osteotomies,[5,15,27] although such correction may not occur at the apex of the forefoot deformity.

More proximal osteotomies have been described and provide a correction at the apex of the deformity.[28–30] Such an osteotomy allows correction by derotating, dorsiflexing, and abducting the forefoot. A crescenteric osteotomy enables a simpler deformity correction by rotating the forefoot about an axis, although it is technically more difficult to create the osteotomy itself. Creating a multiplanar closing wedge osteotomy using straight cuts is simpler to perform, with the drawback of being more difficult to accurately correct the deformity. In 1968, Japas[30] described a dorsally based closing wedge midfoot osteotomy. This osteotomy was combined with a Steindler release of the plantar fascia to allow compression at the osteotomy and had the advantage of being performed through the apex of the deformity. Wicart and Seringe[26] have published the results of a plantar opening edge osteotomy of the 3 cuneiform bones. The investigators describe this osteotomy as providing a "real

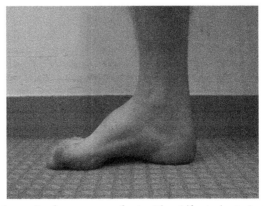

Fig. 4. Clinical photograph of a cavovarus foot with midfoot plantaris deformity.

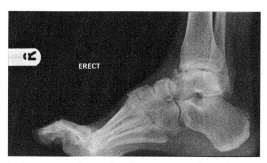

Fig. 5. Lateral weight-bearing radiograph of a cavovarus foot demonstrating the apex of the midfoot plantaris deformity through the cuneiform and cuboid bones.

detwisting of the helicoidal deformity." Mubarak and Van Valin[15] describe a stepwise series of midfoot osteotomies, including a closing wedge osteotomy of the first metatarsal, an opening plantar wedge osteotomy of the medial cuneiform, a cuboid closing wedge osteotomy, and lesser metatarsal osteotomies as required. The reasoning behind this series of operations was obtaining an accurate correction of the cavus deformity while maintaining forefoot mobility.

The aim of any midfoot or forefoot osteotomy is to obtain union across the osteotomy site and achieve a balanced forefoot. To do this, the osteotomy should ideally be performed at the apex of any deformity and allow correction in all planes. As a consequence, the senior author most frequently performs an osteotomy through the cuneiforms and the cuboid that allows the forefoot to be dorsiflexed, abducted, and supinated (**Figs. 6** and **7**).

SOFT-TISSUE RELEASES
Plantar Fascia Release

The need for a plantar fascia release is debatable and variable in the literature. During correction of the cavovarus foot, a plantar fascia release may be performed in all cases,[4,5,12,18,20,22,24,25,30,31] as a selective procedure,[15,23,26,27] or rarely.[21] The plantar fascia is understood to play a major role in foot biomechanics during gait as described by the Windlass mechanism. As a consequence of the attachment of the plantar fascia to the heel and the base of the toes, its division automatically increases the distal

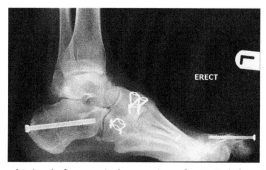

Fig. 6. Radiographs obtained after surgical correction of a CMT deformity showing a calcaneal osteotomy, midfoot osteotomies through the cuneiform and cuboid bones, and a Jones procedure of the hallux.

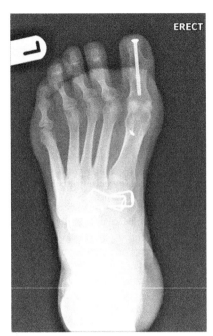

Fig. 7. Radiograph of a foot after a Jones procedure. In this case, a suture anchor has been used to fix the EHL tendon to the neck of the first metatarsal.

progression of the fat pad and the clawing of the toes. It is the authors' belief that correction of the foot deformity in a stepwise manner results in a plantar fascia release being rarely required. This procedure primarily involves correction of the pronated forefoot and the hyperextension of the toes. If the forefoot and toes are reduced, the plantar fascia moves proximally, reducing the inverting force on the calcaneum. In addition, it is thought that preservation of the fascia is of paramount importance in enabling normal foot biomechanics during the gait cycle after surgical correction of the foot deformity. A plantar fascia release is considered if a midfoot osteotomy remains distracted dorsally by an intact fascial band on the plantar aspect, which is not necessary in most cases. If undertaken, it is obligatory to correct the claw toes and hold them in the corrected position.

Tendoachilles Lengthening

The tendoachilles must be carefully assessed. If an equinus contracture is evident and causing deformity, then this must be surgically addressed to enable a planti-grade foot. If such a contracture is evident, this may require either a lengthening of the tendoachilles or more a proximal gastrocnemius recession if the soleus is spared.[4,8,20,22,24,30] The factors that need to be carefully considered when assessing the need for a tendoachilles lengthening (TAL) are the ability to dorsiflex the ankle to neutral, the calcaneal pitch, and the heel position. A midfoot plantaris deformity must not be confused with an equinus deformity at the ankle, and this can be differentiated radiologically by the inclination of the talus. If the heel is in varus, the increased calcaneal pitch is a consequence of rotation of the calcaneum and a TAL aids in correction of this. If the heel is in neutral, the increased calcaneal pitch is likely secondary to longstanding calf weakness and a TAL should be avoided.

Occasionally, a tight tendoachilles is associated with knee hyperextension and quadriceps weakness. In this situation, care must be taken not to overlengthen the gastrosoleus complex, as this may exacerbate knee weakness and result in instability. If the calcaneus has a high pitch, it usually means that the cavus foot is essentially in the foot. Great care must be made to differentiate this from the apparent increased pitch created by the varus heel position. Lengthening of the calf complex in the calcaneus deformity predictably produces severe calf weakness and can make walking difficult. In addition, overlengthening is also difficult to correct.

TENDON TRANSFERS
Peroneus Longus to Brevis Transfer

Tendon transfers are certainly required to obtain a balanced foot. The deforming forces are the result of an imbalance between agonist and antagonists, and these imbalances need to be addressed to prevent fixed deformities developing. Peroneus longus remains strong and produces forefoot pronation[7,15,20,21,25,32] by driving the cuboid under the navicular, causing rotation through the midfoot. A peroneus longus to peroneus brevis transfer acts to reduce the deforming force of peroneus longus and strengthen the eversion force of peroneus brevis. This transfer can be performed over the lateral aspect of the calcaneum using the same oblique incision through which the calcaneal osteotomy is performed. Peroneus longus is divided distally in the incision, proximal to the cuboid tunnel. The peroneal tubercle, which lies between the tendons on the lateral calcaneal wall is excised, and a longus to brevis tenodesis is performed. The authors' favored technique is using a Pulvertaft weave.

Tibialis Posterior Tendon Transfer

If the deforming force of a strong tibialis posterior is causing inversion and plantar flexion, this tendon is transferred to the lateral border of the foot via the interosseous membrane,[6–8,21] which also aids a relatively weak tibialis anterior and reduces the recruitment of the long toe extensors in assisting in ankle dorsiflexion. In addition, reducing the recruitment of the long toe extensors has a beneficial impact on the lesser toe deformities, which is another reason to avoid transferring the long toe extensors to the metatarsal necks (as will be discussed later). Due to the intact flexor hallucis longus and flexor digitorum longus, active inversion of the hindfoot is maintained. It is preferable to overlateralize the tibialis posterior tendon attachment to the dorsum of the foot than have a recurrence of the inversion deformity at a later date. In rare circumstances in which the tibialis anterior remains reasonably strong, peroneus tertius has some action, but the longus and brevis are profoundly weak, the tibialis posterior can be taken behind the ankle and transferred to the peroneii. If tibialis anterior is also weak (Medical Research Council [MRC] grading 3/5), a further option is to transfer tibialis posterior to the dorsolateral foot through the interosseous membrane to aid ankle dorsiflexion. In this situation, the authors would also perform a peroneus longus to brevis tenodesis so that any residual activity in these muscles produces an everting force.

Tibialis Anterior Tendon Transfer

A further option to correct the inversion forces is to transfer the tibialis anterior rather than the tibialis posterior tendon to the lateral aspect of the foot.[4,24,25,31] This correction must be performed only if the tibialis anterior muscle maintains power of MRC grading 4 or 5 and therefore continues to act as an active inverter of the hindfoot.

Due to the potential active involvement of tibialis anterior in the disease process, there are concerns over the efficacy of this transfer over time.[31] It is the authors' belief that a tibialis posterior tendon transfer remains a more reliable option.

TOE DEFORMITIES
Jones Procedure

Clawing of the hallux requires a combined soft-tissue and bony procedure. The deformity is a consequence of a weak tibialis anterior, necessitating the recruitment of EHL for ankle dorsiflexion. In addition, intrinsic muscle weakness allows relative overactivity of the long flexor acting on the distal phalanx. A modified Jones procedure corrects both a flexible or fixed deformity, with a rerouting of the EHL tendon through the first metatarsal neck and arthrodesis of the IP joint (see **Figs. 6** and **7**).[5,12,21,22,24,25,33] Transferring the long extensor tendon proximally allows continued recruitment of the EHL muscle to aid ankle dorsiflexion, an action that also actively elevates the first metatarsal. In addition, correcting the dorsiflexion deformity of the hallux both reduces the plantar flexion force on the first metatarsal head and prevents the exacerbation of the cavus deformity through the windlass mechanism. This combined procedure must be performed secondarily to any midfoot procedures, as a corrective midfoot osteotomy shortens the dorsal bony architecture and subsequently reduces the tension of the extensor tendons. Tensioning of the extensor tendon transfer must therefore be performed after any such bony procedures.

Flexor to Extensor Tendon Transfer

After correction of the forefoot deformity by performing the appropriate osteotomies, the plantar fascia is pulled proximally as the length of the medial longitudinal arch increases (and height decreases). Due to the distal attachment of the plantar fascia to the plantar plate of the proximal phalanges, the phalanges correct from their hyperextended position and provide some degree of correction of the claw toe deformities. If this is not sufficient and the toes remain mobile, flexor to extensor tendon transfers may be performed to further improve the position of the toes[4,12,20,24]; this is also the case if a release of the plantar fascia has been performed. Once toe deformities have become fixed, a proximal IP joint arthrodesis or excision arthroplasty is required.

Extensor Tendon Transfers

Transferring the long extensors of the lesser toes proximally to the metatarsal shaft reduces the clawing deformity of the toes and assists a weakened tibialis anterior in ankle dorsiflexion. To achieve this, the extensor digitorum tendons are transferred to metatarsal necks[7] or the cuneiforms.[8,21,24,32]

The authors prefer to avoid a transfer of the long extensor tendons from the lesser toes to the metatarsal necks. Although the long extensors are a deforming force in the intrinsic minus foot, a transfer of these tendons leaves the toes unable to counterbalance the deforming force of the long flexor tendons. If one combines correction of the medial longitudinal arch with long-extensor tendon transfers to the metatarsal necks, one can overcorrect the toe deformities, with resultant flexion deformities at the proximal and distal IP joints. This dynamic deformity is difficult to correct.

THE SURGICAL PLAN

The order in which surgery is performed is important, as corrective osteotomies influence the effect that the overlying soft tissues have. In addition, forefoot and midfoot surgeries may obviate additional hindfoot realignment. The fixed forefoot deformity is addressed first, with either a dorsiflexion osteotomy of the first metatarsal or a more extensive midfoot derotation osteotomy. After forefoot correction, a valgising osteotomy should be performed if required. On completion of bony surgery, soft-tissue balancing is completed, which may involve multiple procedures, and usually always necessitates a peroneus longus to brevis transfer. Other procedures may include a tibialis posterior transfer and a tendoachilles procedure. If residual toe deformities are present, these are then corrected as a final step. Often the initial flexible toe deformities are improved after the more proximal surgery, and the authors believe these are best undertreated if there is any debate that corrective surgery may still be required. This surgery takes time and sometimes seems almost too much at one sitting, but in general it is better to get maximum control at the time of surgery rather than leave an unpredictable consequence of an undertreated deformity.

OUTCOMES OF SURGERY

As concluded by Holmes and Hansen[34] in their review article in 1993, "Results of surgical procedures are difficult to evaluate and compare largely because of the variety and combinations of procedures, as well as the lack of uniformity in outcome criteria." This conclusion continues to be the situation. The historical literature also includes surgery for the correction of the cavovarus foot resulting from multiple etiologies.[5,15,23,26,27] Due to the unique muscle imbalances resulting in the deformity in patients with CMT disease, this condition must ideally be reviewed in isolation to obtain any meaningful results.

In 1984, Gould[12] published the results of 18 feet in 10 patients with CMT disease. The corrective surgery comprised a radical plantar fascia release, lateral closing wedge calcaneal osteotomy, basal osteotomies of the metatarsals, and a Jones procedure. Foot correction was maintained at 3- to 6-year review, and patients were pleased with the outcome of the surgery. Roper and Tibrewal[24] published their results in 1989, with 10 patients reviewed at 14 years. Procedures performed included a plantar fascia release, calcaneal osteotomy, a Jones procedure, and a tibialis anterior tendon transfer. Two patients had required further surgery, but no subsequent triple arthrodeses were performed. Outcome was reported as "good" in all patients using the outcome scoring system defined by Levitt and colleagues.[22]

Wicart and Seringe[26] published results on the surgical correction of pes cavovarus in children, with 16 of the 26 patients included diagnosed with CMT disease. Surgery included a plantar fascia release, a plantar opening wedge osteotomy of the cuneiforms, a first metatarsal osteotomy, and a Dwyer calcaneal osteotomy. In these 16 patients, 8 of the 26 feet operated on had undergone a triple arthrodesis at a mean of 6.9 years.

A long-term follow-up of 25 patients (41 feet) with CMT disease was reviewed at a mean of 26 years.[25] Reconstruction consisted of a first metatarsal osteotomy, a peroneus longus tendon transfer, a plantar fascia release, a Jones procedure, and a selective tibialis anterior tendon transfer. No subsequent triple arthrodeses were performed, and 11 of 41 feet had evidence of moderate to severe osteoarthritis. The investigators concluded that this rate of degenerative changes within the foot and ankle complex was lower than the reported rate following triple arthrodesis. Leeuwesteijn and colleagues[21] reported the midterm results of 33 patients (52 feet) at a mean of 57 months. Patients underwent a first metatarsal osteotomy, a calcaneal osteotomy if required, and tendon transfers in the form of peroneus longus and tibialis posterior tendon transfers. Two patients required a subsequent triple arthrodesis, and 90% of patients were satisfied after surgery.

The difficulty in obtaining a plantigrade and balanced foot using joint sparing surgery must not be underestimated. A pedobarographic study by Chan and colleagues[35] found foot pressure distribution after surgery was not normalized, despite significant improvements in all radiographic parameters. The investigators concluded that patients must be counseled as to the possibility of persistent symptoms after corrective surgery. They believe that outcome of surgery is not based on correction of the various radiographic parameters but more importantly on achieving a balanced foot; this requires a foot to be rotationally stable (no residual forefoot pronation), plantigrade through the ankle, and with a corrected heel position. If a residual cavus deformity remains but the above-mentioned criteria are met, the patient is more likely to have a good outcome compared with that of a foot that is fully corrected but not adequately balanced. If the only way to achieve a balanced and plantigrade foot is a triple arthrodesis, then this option needs to be carefully considered.

SUMMARY

Foot deformity in the patient with CMT disease frequently presents in the young patient, with symptoms such as abnormal gait, forefoot pain, ankle instability, and changing foot posture. Due to the poor outcomes associated with both nonoperative management and triple arthrodesis, joint sparing surgery is the preferable treatment option. Numerous surgical procedures have been described, all with the aim of achieving a plantigrade and balanced foot. The surgery must be tailored to the requirements of the individual patient and involves a combination of soft-tissue releases, tendon transfers, and osteotomies. The outcomes reported in the literature are variable, but suggest that joint sparing surgery in the young patient with CMT disease is a viable and a preferable alternative to triple arthrodesis.

REFERENCES

1. Charcot JM, Marie P. Sur une forme particuliere d'atrophie musculaire progressive, souvent familiale debutant par les pieds et les jambs et atteignant plus tard les mains. Revue Medicale Paris 1886;6:97–138.
2. Tooth HH. The peroneal type of progressive muscular atrophy [dissertation]. London: HK Lewis; 1886.
3. Krajewski KM, Lewis RA, Fuerst DR, et al. Neurological dysfuction and axonal degeneration in Charcot-Marie-Tooth disease type 1A. Brain 2000;123:1516–27.
4. Jacobs JE, Carr CR. Progressive muscular atrophy of the peroneal type. Orthopaedic management and end result study. J Bone Joint Surg Am 1950;32:27–38.
5. Sammarco GJ, Taylor R. Cavovarus foot treated with combined calcaneus and metatarsal osteotomies. Foot Ankle Int 2001;22:19–30.
6. Wukich DK, Bowen JR. A long-term study of triple arthrodesis for correction of pes cavovarus in Charcot-Marie-Tooth disease. J Pediatr Orthop 1989;9:433–7.
7. Wetmore RS, Drennan JC. Long-term results of triple arthrodesis in Charcot-Marie-Tooth disease. J Bone Joint Surg Am 1989;71:417–22.
8. Mann DC, Hsu JD. Triple arthrodesis in the treatment of fixed cavovarus foot deformity in adolescent patients with Charcot-Marie-Tooth disease. Foot Ankle 1992;13:1–6.
9. Mann RA, Missirian J. Pathophysiology of Charcot-Marie-Tooth disease. Clin Orthop Relat Res 1988;(234):221–8.

10. Tynan MC, Klenerman L, Helliwell TR, et al. Investigation of muscle imbalance in the leg in symptomatic forefoot pes cavus: a mulitdiscipinary study. Foot Ankle 1992;13:489–500.
11. Gallardo E, Garcia A, Combarros O, et al. Charcot-Marie-Tooth disease type 1A duplication: spectrum of clinical and magnetic resonance imaging features in leg and foot muscles. Brain 2006;129:426–37.
12. Gould N. Surgery in advanced Charcot Marie Tooth disease. Foot Ankle 1984;4: 267–73.
13. Krause FG, Henning J, Pfander G, et al. Cavovaris foot realignment to treat anteromedial ankle arthrosis. Foot Ankle Int 2013;34:54–64.
14. Coleman SS, Chesnut WJ. A simple test for hindfoot flexibility in the cavovarus foot. Clin Orthop Relat Res 1977;123:60–2.
15. Mubarak SJ, Van Valin SE. Osteotomies of the foot for the cavus deformities in childen. J Pediatr Orthop 2009;29:294–9.
16. Price BD, Price CT. A simple demonstration of hindfoot flexibility in the cavovarus foot. J Pediatr Orthop 1997;17:18–9.
17. Dwyer FC. Osteotomy of the calcaneum for pes cavus. J Bone Joint Surg Am 1959;41:80–6.
18. Samilson RL. Cresentic osteotomy of the os calcis for calcaneocavus feet. In: Bateman JE, editor. Foot science. Philadelphia: WB Saunders; 1976. p. 18–25.
19. Knupp M, Pagenstert G, Valderrabano V, et al. Osteotomies in varus malalignment of the ankle. Oper Orthop Traumatol 2008;20:262–73.
20. Alexander IJ, Johnson KA. Assessment and management of pes cavus in Charcot-Marie-Tooth disease. Clin Orthop Relat Res 1989;246:273–81.
21. Leeuwesteijn AE, de Visser E, Louwerens JW. Flexible cavovarus feet in Charcot-Marie-Tooth disease treated with first ray proximal dorsiflexion osteotomy combined with soft tissue surgery: a short-term to mid-term study. Foot Ankle Surg 2010;16:142–7.
22. Levitt RL, Canale ST, Cooke AJ, et al. The role of foot surgery in progressive neuromuscular disorders in children. J Bone Joint Surg Am 1973;55: 1396–410.
23. Paulos L, Coleman SS, Samuelson KM. Pes cavovarus. Review of a surgical approach using selective soft-tissue procedures. J Bone Joint Surg Am 1980; 62:942–53.
24. Roper BA, Tibrewal SB. Soft tissue surgery in Charcot Marie Tooth disease. J Bone Joint Surg Am 1989;71:17–20.
25. Ward CM, Dolan LA, Bennett DL, et al. Long-term results of reconstruction for treatment of a flexible cavovarus foot in Charcot-Marie-Tooth disease. J Bone Joint Surg Am 2008;90:2632–42.
26. Wicart P, Seringe R. Plantar opening-wedge osteotomy of cuneiform bones combined with selective plantar release and Dwyer osteotomy for pes cavovarus in children. J Pediatr Orthop 2006;26:100–8.
27. Watanabe RS. Metatarsal osteotomy for the cavovarus foot. Clin Orthop Relat Res 1990;252:217–30.
28. Jahss MH. Tarsometatarsal truncated wedge arthrodesis for pes cavus and equinovarus deformity of the fore part of the foot. J Bone Joint Surg Am 1980; 62:713–22.
29. Wilcox PG, Weiner DS. The Akron midtarsal dome osteotomy in the treatment of rigid pes cavus: a preliminary review. J Pediatr Orthop 1985;5:333–8.
30. Japas L. Surgical treatment of pes cavus by tarsal V-osteotomy. Preliminary report. J Bone Joint Surg Am 1968;50:927–44.

31. Shapiro F, Bresnan MJ. Orthopaedic management of childhood neuromuscular disease. Part II: peripheral neuropathies, Friedrich's ataxia, and arthrogryposis multiles congenital. J Bone Joint Surg Am 1982;64:949–53.
32. Cole WH. The treatment of the claw foot. J Bone Joint Surg Am 1940;23:895–908.
33. Jones R, Lovett RW. Orthopaedic surgery. London: Henry Frowde and Hodder & Stoughton; 1923.
34. Holmes JR, Hansen ST Jr. Foot and ankle manifestations of Chacot-Marie-Tooth disease. Foot Ankle 1993;14:476–86.
35. Chan G, Sampath J, Miller F, et al. The role of the dynamic pedobarograph in assessing treatment of cavovarus feet in children with Charcot-Marie-Tooth disease. J Pediatr Orthop 2007;27:510–6.

What is the Role of Tendon Transfer in the Cavus Foot?

Martin Huber, MD

KEYWORDS

- Cavus foot • Tendon transfer • Muscle imbalance • Neuropathic foot disorder

KEY POINTS

- Cavus and cavovarus deformities of the hindfoot as a result of muscle imbalance caused by a neuropathic disorder need surgical treatment if not responding to shoe modification and orthoses.
- The agonist–antagonist equilibrium is conditio sine qua non for a good long-term result.
- Bony procedures and arthrodeses can only withstand if muscle balance is re-established.
- The overpowering flexors and invertors need to be redirected to substitute for the weak extensors and evertors.

PATHOMECHANICAL CONSIDERATIONS

Different patterns of muscle imbalance can lead to deviation of the subtalar joint complex and hence to hindfoot varus and cavovarus deformity. Depending on the power and the insertion of the muscles in question, the resulting action leads to different malposition of hind- and midfoot. Any imbalance between agonist/antagonist muscular forces will lead to a relative overpower of one or the other muscle action causing malalignment and deformity.

Whereas the acquired planovalgus deformity is typically the result of an incompetency of the posterior tibial tendon, cavovarus deformity, whether rigid or flexible is usually caused by neurologic disorders. Hereditary sensory motor neuropathy is the most common etiology of a bilateral cavovarus deformity. Due to its progressive character, it is a prototype of manifestation of the neuropathic cavovarus foot. While flexible in early stages, the affected foot becomes more and more rigid over time.

Three important pairs of agonist/antagonist muscles determine hind- and midfoot motion. Inversion/eversion is controlled by the interplay of posterior tibial muscle and peroneus brevis muscle, as well as the reciprocal action of peroneus longus muscle and anterior tibial muscle. Controlled dorsiflexion/plantarflexion of the foot and ankle is a result of the interaction between anterior tibial muscle and gastrocnemius–soleus complex. Forefoot deformity, such as progressive claw toe deformity,

Department for Foot and Ankle surgery, Schulthess Klinik, CH-8008 Zürich, Switzerland
E-mail address: martin.huber@bluewin.ch

Foot Ankle Clin N Am 18 (2013) 689–695
http://dx.doi.org/10.1016/j.fcl.2013.08.002
1083-7515/13/$ – see front matter © 2013 Elsevier Inc. All rights reserved.

foot.theclinics.com

is rather determined by imbalanced inter-relation of intrinsic and extrinsic muscle forces.

Although a weakness of the peroneus longus is usually not present in hereditary sensory motor neuropathy, the peroneus brevis muscle and the anterior tibialis muscle are primarily affected with progressive weakness.[1] Dysfunction of the intrinsic muscles will follow.[2]

Weakness of the peroneus brevis results in unopposed action of the posterior tibial muscle as its antagonist leading to inversion of the hindfoot. Overpowering through peroneus longus and gastrocnemius–soleus are the result of the weakness of anterior tibial muscle. Because of its insertion at the plantar aspect of the base of the first metatarsal peroneus longus, action leads to hyperflexion of the first metatarsal.

Further deformities are the result of the previously mentioned primary causes; because of hindfoot inversion, the Achilles tendon will shift medially and act as a secondary invertor. This circumstance will accentuate the deforming forces and increase a tendency towards contracture. Recruiting extensor hallucis longus and extensor digitorum longus as secondary ankle dorsiflexors will lead to cock-up deformity of the hallux and clawtoe deformity of the lesser toes. The plantarflexed first metatarsal and the lesser metatarsals will further be depressed by the dorsally contracted and subluxed metatarso-phalangeal joints. Additional contracture of the plantar fascia will accentuate the windlass mechanism and further depress the metatarsal heads, holding the forefoot in adduction and inverting the calcaneus.

CLINICAL EVALUATION

The specific gait pattern and static deformity of the cavus foot with high arch, hindfoot varus and adducted midfoot confirm the global diagnosis. A proper evaluation with consecutive decision making for a specific treatment can then only be done by thorough examination with the patient sitting with hanging lower leg. The Coleman block test is of high didactical value to demonstrate the so-called forefoot-driven flexible cavus deformity. However, the surgeon must be able to manually demonstrate the same maneuver in the nonweight-bearing foot by holding the heel and the Achilles in the palm of the hand and applying valgus stress. The flexible hindfoot will reduce, and as a consequence, rotate the forefoot into pronation. Later, on the operating table, this manipulation will be the only possible technique to quantify any achieved correction of the hindfoot, whereas the correction of forefoot pronation can be assessed with a plate under the foot to simulate weight bearing.

With regard to a functional realignment with tendon transfer, the careful assessment of strength and function of all agonist/antagonist muscles pairs stands in the center of the clinical examination. Only by identifying the deforming forces can surgery be planned correctly.[3]

SURGICAL TREATMENT

The goals of surgery should be a balanced and plantigrade foot to improve function and to avoid late sequelae such as varus instability of the ankle, overload symptoms in the mid- and forefoot or hammertoe deformities with dislocation of the MP joints.

Timing of surgery is dependent on age and severity of the deformity and its etiology. Although a static neurologic deficit with mild symptoms often is treated with shoe modifications, inserts, and physical therapy, for progressive symptomatic deformities, an early surgical treatment must be considered, because soft tissue procedures at an early stage seem to postpone the need for a triple arthrodesis.[4–6]

Fixed deformities usually can only be corrected by performing fusions and osteot-omies. In many cases, a triple arthrodesis is indicated. Whether fusions of the peritalar joints or osteotomies are being performed to statically correct a deformity, a dynamic balance with tendon transfer or tendon resection with soft tissue release is prerequi-site to maintain a successful result over time. If imbalance of the deforming forces (ie, in many cases the posterior tibial muscle) is neglected, progressive deformity distal to the fusion site will recur.[3,7] Flexible cavus foot treatment, however, does not require a hindfoot arthrodesis, with soft tissue release, tendon transfer, and osteotomies considered the preferred management.

To re-establish the equilibrium between an overpowering muscle and its antagonist, basically 2 different approaches are conceivable. The first would be to redirect the stronger partner in order to weaken its intrinsic function and partially substitute the lost activity of the weak antagonist. The other option in many cases can also be the weakening by elongation or the resection of the deforming muscle–tendon unit, espe-cially in a severe case in which a poor result with limited function and minimal postre-habilitation range of movement must be expected. This second procedure is mostly indicated in conjunction with hindfoot fusion or in low-demand patients.

THE PRINCIPLES OF TENDON TRANSFER

Some prerequisites for a successful active muscle balancing must be considered carefully when planning a tendon transfer. Furthermore, the patient must understand the rationale behind the transfer and what he or she can expect from the surgery. Two main purposes of the tendon transfer are intended. The first is to eliminate any deform-ing force by harvesting (ie, cutting) the tendon from its insertion; the second is to augment the weak function by rerouting that same tendon muscle unit. Basic consid-erations about tendon transfer are listed:

- The tendon to be transferred ideally should be phasic (ie, work in the same direc-tion like the function unit to be substitute). The rehabilitation will be much easier, as there is not a completely new function to learn.
- An adequate range of movement within the joint on which the transferred muscle will act should be remaining if the transfer is being utilized to correct the defor-mity. It is of paramount importance, however, to understand that even in a fixed cavovarus with the need for a triple arthrodesis, a balance of any deforming forces must be re-established. With that in mind, the range of movement is of a secondary role.
- To accomplish the goal of a dynamically working tendon transfer, the muscle must have adequate power. It is a fact that muscle will lose at least 1 grade of po-wer with the transfer. In general, therefore, it is recommended to transfer only muscle tendon units with a power of M4 or M5. Ryssman and Myerson point out that even a weak muscle with only minimal power will lead to a long-term deformity and can be one of the reasons for recurrent deformity. Therefore they recommend the transfer even for a weak muscle if it is considered to be the deforming force.[3] In the author's hands, this will apply in cases in which a simultaneous fusion is planned, as well as in the flexible deformity, in which the aim is to balance the forces. In these cases, the patient needs to be well informed about the goal of the operation, and expectations need to be clarified in advance.
- After the transfer, the tendon should run in a straight course. Acute angulation or kinking should be avoided. This concern is especially important when transfer-ring the posterior tibial muscle through the interosseus membrane to the dorsum of the foot.

- Fixation can be achieved through a bone tunnel or with a suture anchor for direct tendon-to-bone healing. An indirect fixation with side-to-side tenodesis is usually performed when transferring the peroneus longus to the peroneus brevis tendon. A stable fixation is important to allow an early rehabilitation program with passive and active range-of-movement exercises.

TENDON TRANSFERS

As mentioned before, balancing muscular strength in the cavovarus foot is crucial. Most of the time, an additional static alignment with soft tissue release and osteotomies or fusions is required. Technically, it is advisable to perform this soft tissue release as the first step, followed by osteotomies or fusions. Where harvesting the tendon from its deviating insertional point is part of the soft tissue release, rerouting and tensioning are typically done only after the static alignment has been achieved. The peroneus longus-to-brevis transfer, the posterior tibial transfers, the anterior tibial tendon transfer, and the extensor hallucis longus and extensor digitorum longus transfers are the major transfers most often used. These common tendon transfers will be discussed in detail.

Peroneus Longus-to-Brevis Tendon Transfer

Chronic lateral ankle instability will often recur if the underlying pathology is not recognized and treated adequately. One of the causes of recurrent twisting injury is a cavovarus alignment of the hindfoot. In cases with an overpowering peroneus longus muscle, the typical picture of the forefoot driven cavovarus deformity presents. Because of its insertion onto the plantar aspect of the base of the first metatarsal, the peroneus longus muscle acts primarily as a flexor to the first metatarsal, causing a pronation of the forefoot. As a consequence, the hindfoot turns into varus. Hypercallosity under the lateral border of the foot and under the MP 1 joint and the head of the first metatarsal will be a regular finding in these patients. Chronic ankle instability may be noted, and fatigue fractures of the fifth metatarsal can be late sequelae. In the common forms of hereditary sensory motor neuropathy, the peroneus longus muscle is among the strongest deforming forces.

The transfer of the peroneus longus to brevis seems to be the most common transfer in those cases of idiopathic cavus feet, where the maximal advantage is achieved in a young population with flexible deformity.[8] It allows the first metatarsal to extend and reinforces the weak eversion of the hindfoot at the same time.

Other indications for the peroneus longus transfer are the symptomatic cavus deformity with the characteristic overpowering of the peroneus longus muscle over a weak anterior tibial muscle and in medial contractures with an overpowering posterior tibial muscle. In these conditions, the peroneus longus transfer is only part of a complex rebalancing with additional tendon transfers. Its contribution will still be to augment the eversion forces and work against the normal power of the posterior tibial muscle as well as it will help to balance the weak anterior tibial muscle.

Technically, the transfer is performed through a lateral incision over the distal course of the peroneals and extended over the base of the fifth metatarsal. If a calcaneal osteotomy is performed at the same time, the transfer can also be achieved through that same L-incision. The peroneus longus tendon is transected under the cuboid. An often existing accessory os peroneale is resected. In this distal area, the peroneus longus and the peroneus brevis run in separate sheaths. The peroneal tubercle is removed so that the longus can be swung to the brevis, where it is sutured side-to-side in neutral hindfoot position. As one must deal with a hyperactive function of the peroneus longus muscle, it is usually not indicated to pretension it prior to tenodesis. As an alternative technique, it might be easier to perform the tenodesis in neutral hindfoot position before the distal tenotomy. In chronic ankle instability, the peroneus brevis tendon can present with chronic longitudinal tears. If this is the case, a longer running suture to perform the tenodesis is sometimes needed. A direct insertion of the peroneus longus onto the base of the fifth metatarsal using a bone anchor can be considered also.

Other indications for a peroneus longus transfer may be to reinforce not only foot eversion but also dorsiflexion power by rerouting it to the lateral cuneiform on the dorsum of the foot or reinsertion onto the calcaneus in a case of a weak triceps surae.[9]

Posterior Tibial Tendon Transfer

Dysfunction of the peroneus brevis muscle will allow the posterior tibial muscle to act unopposed; foot inversion and progressive contracture of the medial soft tissues will be the result. The goal of the transfer of the posterior tibial tendon is to first weaken the deforming power and then to strengthen deficient functions of the foot.

The most challenging transfer is that to the dorsum of the foot to substitute for a weak anterior tibial tendon. This situation commonly occurs in hereditary sensory motor neuropathy. To achieve this goal, the tendon must be rerouted behind the tibia through the interosseus membrane to the dorsum of the foot, usually to the intermediate cuneiform. Although technically demanding, it will also require a longer period of rehabilitation. By transferring the posterior tibial tendon to the dorsum of the foot, it will no longer act as a flexor but now as an extensor muscle on the ankle. This nonphasic function will necessarily lead to a reduction of strength.

The modified 4-incision technique published by Hsu and Hoffer[10] in 1978 is now the most popular technique for the interosseous transfer. Harvesting as much length of the posterior tibial tendon from its insertion as possible is important. Through this first incision, a medial release of the contracted structures can be performed (ie, the plantar fascia and spring ligament). The tendon is then mobilized into a second incision posteromedial to the tibia at the level of the musculotendinous junction. In order to avoid a later kinking of the transferred tendon, it is important to perform this incision high enough, approximately 15 to 20 cm proximal to the ankle. The tendon is then passed directly behind the tibia. Care must be taken to pass it medial to the neurovascular bundle with the deep peroneal nerve. The third incision to expose the interosseous membrane is performed anterolaterally to the tibia at a level approximately 7 to 10 cm above the joint line. The interosseous membrane must be split and partially excised to allow unrestricted passage of the posterior tibial tendon. A clamp is then passed from the anterolateral border of the tibia around the posterior face into the medial incision where the tendon can be grasped and pulled anteriorly. Doing so, even the tibial nerve is safe during the whole procedure. From here the tendon is passed subcutaneously to the dorsum of the foot into the fourth incision. The subcutaneous transfer is preferable to a transfer under the extensor retinaculum; usually the length of the posterior tibial tendon will not allow the longer passage underneath, and the resulting vector of strength is more favorable due to the resulting bowstringing. Insertion onto the second cuneiform will provide a neutral dorsiflexion, whereas insertion onto the third cuneiform or the cuboid will also help to improve foot eversion. To find the isometric point for ideal placement of tendon insertion, the shape of the foot must be taken into consideration. Where in the normally aligned foot the ideal insertion is frequently onto the intermediate cuneiform, for the cavus foot center of rotation is regularly more lateral.

Where the deforming force of the posterior tibial muscle is causing an isolated deviation of the hindfoot into adductovarus in a deficiency of the peroneals with intact strength of the anterior tibial muscle, a phasic transfer of the posterior tibial tendon onto the peroneus brevis tendon can be performed. Either a split or complete transfer behind the tibia is possible.[3]

Anterior Tibial Tendon Transfer

Where deformity is caused by overpowering activity of the anterior tibial muscle leading to midfoot adduction/supination and accentuating the cavus deformity, transfer of the anterior tibial tendon to the second or third cuneiform can help to rebalance the foot. Even if the anterior tibial muscle is weak, in many cases it will still contribute to the deformity and may be a reason for persistent deformity with deterioration over time. If strength is still maintained, an isolated transfer is performed. In pronounced weakness, augmentation with simultaneous transfer of the long toe extensors is advisable.

In adult reconstruction, a split transfer as used in pediatric surgery in cases of spastic deformities is rarely indicated. A functional complete transfer of the anterior tibial tendon seems to be advantageous over tenodesis with the stirrup.

Extensor Hallucis Longus and Extensor Digitorum Longus Transfers

Weakness of the anterior tibial muscle leads to recruiting of extensor hallucis and extensor digitorum muscles in order to improve dorsiflexion to the ankle. With time, this excessive pull of the long toe extensors will lead to cock-up deformity of the great toe and to claw toe deformities. Cock-up of the great toe causes further depression of the first metatarsal, accentuating the cavus even more. Again, these deviating forces need to be neutralized by transferring them to the midfoot.

The Jones procedure intends to transfer the deforming extensor hallucis longus tendon onto the neck of the first metatarsal. The typically flexed first IP joint is fused. Thus the great toe is no longer forced into dorsiflexion; the force vector that depresses the first metatarsal is relaxed. The extensor hallucis longus now acts as a primary extensor to the first metatarsal, which will decrease the excessive forefoot pronation and the overload symptoms of the MP 1 joint and the sesamoids.

An alternative transfer of the extensor hallucis longus is that to the dorsum of the foot, usually onto the second or third cuneiform. This transfer is often augmented with the simultaneous transfer of the anterior tibial tendon and the extensor digitorum longus also. Despite pronounced weakness of the extensors, it is of greatest importance to bring these deviating forces onto a neutral center as a new insertion point to allow balanced dorsiflexion to the ankle.

SUMMARY

Cavus and cavovarus deformities of the hindfoot as a result of muscle imbalance due to a neuropathic disorder need surgical treatment if not responding to shoe modification and orthoses. The agonist–antagonist equilibrium is conditio sine qua non for a good long-term result. Bony procedures and arthrodeses can only withstand if muscle balance is re-established. The overpowering flexors and invertors need to be redirected to substitute for the weak extensors and evertors.

REFERENCES

1. Hansen ST. The cavovarus/supinated foot deformity and external tibial torsion: the role of the posterior tibial tendon. Foot Ankle Clin 2008;13:325–8.

2. Marks RM. Midfoot and forefoot issues cavovarus foot: assessment and treatment issues. Foot Ankle Clin 2008;13:229–41.
3. Ryssman DB, Myerson MS. Tendon transfers for the adult flexible cavovarus foot. Foot Ankle Clin 2011;16:435–50.
4. Roper BA, Tibrewal SB. Soft tissue surgery in charcot-marie-tooth disease. J Bone Joint Surg Br 1989;71:17–20.
5. Krause F, Wing K, Alastair Y. Neuromuscular issues in cavovarus foot. Foot Ankle Clin 2008;13:243–58.
6. Ward CM, Dolan LA, Bennett DL, et al. Long-term results of reconstruction for treatment of a flexible cavovarus foot in Charcot-Marie-Tooth disease. J Bone Joint Surg Am 2008;90:2631–42.
7. Whetmore R, Drennan J. Long-term results of triple arthrodesis in Charcot-Marie-Tooth disease. J Bone Joint Surg Am 1989;71:417–22.
8. Ortiz C, Wagner E, Keller A. Cavovarus foot reconstruction. Foot Ankle Clin 2009; 14:471–87.
9. Hansen ST. Cavovarus foot (medial peritalar subluxation). In: Hansen ST, editor. Functional reconstruction of the foot and ankle. Philadelphia: Lippincott Williams & Wilkins; 2000. p. 433–5.
10. Hsu J, Hoffer M. Posterior tibial tendon transfer anteriorly through the interosseous membrane: a modification of the technique. Clin Orthop Relat Res 1978; 131:202–4.

What is the Role and Limit of Calcaneal Osteotomy in the Cavovarus Foot?

Jason T. Bariteau, MD[a],*, Brad D. Blankenhorn, MD, MS[b], Josef N. Tofte, BA[c], Christopher W. DiGiovanni, MD[d,e]

KEYWORDS

- Cavovarus foot • Dwyer osteotomy • Lateralizing calcaneal osteotomy
- Z-osteotomy

KEY POINTS

- Hindfoot pathology is commonly seen in patients with cavovarus feet.
- Multiple calcaneal osteotomies have been described to address hindfoot pathology.
- Calcaneal osteotomy not only affects the hindfoot specifically, but alters the biomechanics of the entire foot.
- No clear evidence exists to support one osteotomy over another; the osteotomy chosen should therefore be based on the nature of the desired correction, as well as the surgeon's comfort with any chosen procedure.

INTRODUCTION

Cavus foot deformity, most commonly the result of first-ray plantar flexion, is frequently encountered by the foot and ankle specialist. Over time, an excessively plantar flexed first ray is often compensated by progressive hindfoot varus, leading

Funding Sources: None.
Conflict of Interest: None.
[a] Department of Orthopaedic Surgery, The Warren Alpert Medical School, Brown University, 593 Eddy Street, Providence, RI 02903, USA; [b] Department of Orthopaedics and Rehabilitation, University of New Mexico School of Medicine, UNM Hospitals, MSC 10 8000, 2211 Lomas Boulevard Northeast, 1 University of New Mexico, Albuquerque, NM 87131, USA; [c] Department of Orthopaedic Surgery, The Warren Alpert Medical School, Brown University, Box G-9327, Providence, RI 02912, USA; [d] Foot and Ankle Service, Department of Orthopaedic Surgery, Rhode Island Hospital, The Warren Alpert Medical School, Brown University, 593 Eddy Street, Providence, RI 02903, USA; [e] Department of Orthopaedic Surgery, University Orthopedics, Inc, 100 Butler Drive, Providence, RI 02906, USA
* Corresponding author. Department of Orthopedics, The Warren Alpert Medical School, Brown University, 593 Eddy Street, Providence, RI 02903.
E-mail address: jason.bariteau@gmail.com

Foot Ankle Clin N Am 18 (2013) 697–714
http://dx.doi.org/10.1016/j.fcl.2013.08.001
foot.theclinics.com

to the creation of a cavovarus foot. Cavovarus deformity can be classified by the severity of malalignment ranging from a subtle and flexible cavovarus foot, as described by Manoli and Graham,[1] to a severe cavovarus posture accompanied by fixed bony malalignment. Depending on the magnitude and rigidity of this cavovarus deformity, patients can present with a wide range of complaints. Most commonly, these include lateral forefoot overload, fifth metatarsal fracture, tendinopathy, ankle pain or instability, and metatarsalgia. Generally speaking, one of these problems, rather than the cavovarus deformity itself, will end up driving the patient to seek the attention of a foot and ankle specialist. There are 4 main etiologies that account for most cavovarus foot deformities: neurologic, posttraumatic, residual clubfoot, and idiopathic.[2] The most commonly seen neurologic etiologies include cerebral palsy and Charcot Marie Tooth (CMT) disease.

A cavovarus foot typically presents as a complex relationship between forefoot and hindfoot deformity but can sometimes involve malalignment inherent to the midfoot as well. The epicenter of these deformities can therefore vary greatly as they traverse a broad spectrum of disease, ranging from a truly "subtle" flexible malposition to a seriously imbalanced, rigid, and grotesque malalignment. Regardless of the severity of the deformity and the nature of the presenting complaints, it seems evident from the literature that the calcaneal osteotomy represents one of the most commonly performed surgical mainstays in management. Given the impact that the continuum of cavovarus disease has on timing and severity of presentation, as well as the dearth of substantive evidence regarding what is specifically gained by performing calcaneal osteotomy in such settings, the role of calcaneal osteotomy in treating these deformities remains somewhat ill defined. Although long-standing cavovarus deformity can cause calcaneocuboid and talonavicular joint dysplasia and contracture, for example, the effects of a calcaneal osteotomy on transverse tarsal joint alignment and motion are not well known. In the authors' experience, isolated uniplanar calcaneal osteotomy does not clearly alter the alignment of these joints. Rather, it primarily alters forces transferred from the heel through the tibiotalar joint through alteration of the mechanical axis.[3] However, it is also known that by changing the mechanical alignment of the heel, both the forces and alignment transferred to the forefoot are altered to some extent.[3]

When developing a plan to surgically treat a cavovarus foot, it is useful to determine the significance of the deformity with respect to different regions of the foot. It is important to evaluate the passive correctability level and contribution of deformity across the hindfoot, midfoot, and forefoot. Each of these "independent" regions of the foot can influence the severity and direction of malalignment, and therefore each has described for it specific surgical interventions that can be used for respective corrections. Fortunately, one foot region will often exert significant enough effects across other regions such that these no longer require specific correction based on their ability to passively accommodate after correction of the initial anatomic region. It remains difficult, however, to always predict the ultimate clinical impact of these changes preoperatively, or even intraoperatively in some cases. In general, the nonlengthened calcaneal osteotomy has traditionally been used to treat a symptomatically neutral or varus hindfoot. Although this procedure can impact other parts of the foot (midfoot and forefoot), any residual transverse tarsal joint malposition usually requires joint releases or tendon transfers if the joint remains flexible, and double or triple arthrodesis if it is fixed. Residual forefoot deformity usually requires treatment with a dorsiflexion osteotomy of the first ray or tendon transfers, again depending on the severity of the deformity. Although calcaneal osteotomy is often paramount to optimal cavovarus correction, it is impractical to think that this hindfoot procedure in its purest form can also enact powerful correction through the midfoot or forefoot under most circumstances. Certain exceptions to this may exist, however, and are described later in this article.

TYPES OF CAVUS FEET
Subtle (Mild)

The subtle cavus foot is usually idiopathic in nature. It has been characteristically defined by a plantar flexed first ray.[1] On presentation, most patients may exhibit a flexible hindfoot. Over time, however, the hindfoot can become stiff and rigid.[1] Examination of the patient with subtle cavovarus foot typically reveals a high arch and hindfoot neutrality or subtle varus on standing frontal examination (the heel "peek-a-boo" sign). Coleman block testing is useful in determining the flexibility of the hindfoot and, more specifically, whether or not the hindfoot varus is driven by forefoot valgus. Treatment of the subtle cavovarus foot ranges from nonoperative management with orthotics and physical therapy to operative correction. Any surgical intervention will need to address all presenting symptom generators for the patient, in addition to the underlying foot architecture. Surgery to alter the underlying alignment of a subtle cavovarus foot often includes either forefoot or calcaneal osteotomy.[4] Soft tissue and tendon releases may also be required.

Severe

In contradistinction, a severe cavus foot is often the end product of chronic deformity associated with a plantar flexed first ray, or sometimes even severe plantar flexion through the entire midfoot, an increased calcaneal pitch, and especially neuromuscular foot imbalance (such as seen with CMT). This typically includes a fixed heel varus that no longer corrects with Coleman block testing. Reconstruction of the severe cavus foot invariably requires a complex combination of soft tissue balancing, calcaneal osteotomy, and/or an arthrodesis. Although there are many calcaneal osteotomies described for this purpose, the type that is used is predicated on the nature of desired correction, overall soft tissue tolerance, and the familiarity of the surgeon with the procedure. Other osteotomies may be necessary to correct residual forefoot valgus once appropriate hindfoot valgus is restored.[5]

COMMON CALCANEAL OSTEOTOMIES

There have been multiple calcaneal osteotomies described in the literature for the treatment of hindfoot varus. Many of these were developed for the treatment of deformities resulting from poliomyelitis.[6] The large number of calcaneal osteotomy variations suggests that there exists no singular osteotomy that is ideal for treating all cases of hindfoot varus. The surgeon should therefore be comfortable with performing several different iterations of calcaneal osteotomy to appropriately treat the variable presentations of hindfoot varus. Preoperative use of a hindfoot alignment view, as described by Saltzman and El-Khoury,[7] in conjunction with the Coleman block test, can be useful in deciding the amount of correction that is necessary, and can aid in the decision process for which osteotomy to perform.

The classic osteotomy performed for hindfoot correction of the cavovarus foot has been the Dwyer procedure. The Dwyer osteotomy entails a lateral oblique incision over the tuberosity of the calcaneus. After exposure of the lateral wall of the calcaneus, a lateral closing wedge osteotomy is then performed to address the hindfoot varus.[8] In his 1975 review, Dwyer[8] discussed his experience and highlighted the critical nature of addressing the hindfoot. Further experience with the technique, however, has demonstrated that this osteotomy may not provide sufficient correction for more severe deformity and may also lead to weakening of the Achilles tendon[2] by virtue of shortening heel length. The risk of complications with this procedure is low, however, for a deformity that does not require major correction. The Dwyer osteotomy is still an excellent means for correcting hindfoot varus.

Currently, perhaps the most commonly used osteotomy to address hindfoot varus is the so-called lateralizing calcaneal osteotomy, which can be superiorly translated to correct residual cavus at the same time. This procedure is similarly performed through a lateral approach to calcaneus (**Fig. 1**), after which an oblique linear osteotomy is performed that exits distal to the weight-bearing surface of the tuber. Once the osteotomy is made, the tuberosity can then be translated laterally until sufficient correction of the varus deformity is obtained. If during the tuber manipulation adequate clinical correction, especially superiorly, still remains difficult, complete plantar fascia release from the base of the tuber is recommended. This almost always enables the desired degree of repositioning. The osteotomy is then stabilized with 1 or 2 large screws.[9] With appropriate caution, the neuromuscular risks associated with this osteotomy are believed to be lower than with many of the other osteotomies used to address a varus deformity.[10] Deformity correction, however, is limited to frontal and sagittal plane realignment, and there is a limit to the amount of displacement that can be obtained. This limit has been arbitrarily considered to be approximately 1 cm, although there are few data to support this somewhat dogmatic understanding. To minimize the potential for tarsal tunnel syndrome, nerve impingement, and soft tissue complications, some investigators have advocated either preemptive release of tarsal tunnel or staged reosteotomization of the calcaneus through the same plane for further translational correction, if necessary, based on severity of originating deformity.[11]

Other investigators have investigated performing a posterior displacement osteotomy with superiorization of the tubercle for correction when the primary concern is hindfoot cavus and weak Achilles strength (**Fig. 2**).[12] In the posterior displacement osteotomy, the calcaneus is again approached from a lateral position, and an oblique osteotomy is performed. The tuberosity is then shifted posteriorly and superiorly to improve the moment arm of Achilles and correct the hindfoot cavus. Samilson and Dillin also described a cresentic calcaneal osteotomy for treatment of hindfoot cavus.[13]

In certain situations, many advocate that a single-plane osteotomy cannot provide enough correction.[14] To increase the amount of correction, Pisani[15] described a calcaneal osteotomy, which removed a wedge of bone to specifically augment the effects of both the lateralizing osteotomy and the valgus seen with Dwyer. This was further modified by Malerba and DiMarchi to include a Z-osteotomy that enables similar correction and purportedly less risk to the subtalalar joint.[16] These osteotomy variants add a component of coronal, sagittal, or rotational plane correction (**Fig. 3**).

Knupp and colleagues[14] described a triplanar osteotomy meant to address all aspects of the cavovarus hindfoot (**Fig. 4**). The investigators use a similar scarf-type Z-osteotomy that adds not only a rotational but also a lengthening opportunity when required. The procedure theoretically allows for correction in the frontal, transverse, and sagittal planes. Such an osteotomy is purported to afford a great deal of flexibility for correction of severe deformities, but is technically more difficult to both create as well as fix, and therefore comes with a potentially higher perioperative risk. A larger incision and more dissection are required, increasing the chance of wound problems and injury to adjacent structures, particularly the sural nerve. Due

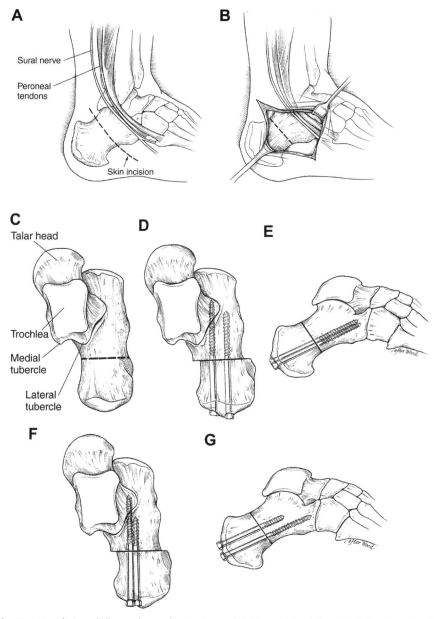

Fig. 1. Lateralizing sliding calcaneal osteotomy. (*A*) A posterior lateral incision is made. (*B*) Once the soft tissues have been retracted, the calcaneus is cut with a saw. (*C*) The medial cut should not penetrate close to the sustentaculum tali. (*D, E*) The osteotomy is held with 2 proximal-distal transcalcaneal screws. (*F, G*) Alternative screw positions. (*Adapted from* Hansen ST Jr, editor. Functional reconstruction of the foot and ankle. Philadelphia: Lippincott Williams and Wilkins; 2000. p. 369; with permission.)

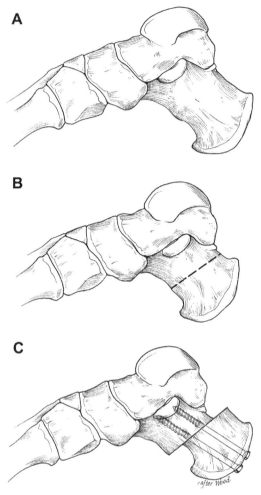

Fig. 2. Posterior calcaneal osteotomy for hindfoot cavus. (*A*) Normal relationship of the hindfoot bones. (*B*) Position of the hindfoot secondary to a weak triceps surae. The osteotomy is made from the lateral aspect. (*C*) The posterior tuberosity fragment is displaced in a dorsal and posterior direction to restore length, reduce the arch, and improve the moment arm of the weak triceps surae muscle. The screws are placed in parallel across the osteotomy site. (*Adapted from* Hansen ST Jr, editor. Functional reconstruction of the foot and ankle. Philadelphia: Lippincott Williams and Wilkins; 2000. p. 373; with permission.)

to the complexity of the osteotomy cuts, unintentional overcorrection has been described.[17]

CALCANEAL OSTEOTOMY INDICATIONS

There are many reports in the literature describing techniques as well as theoretical indications for performing various types of calcaneal osteotomies. Unfortunately, scant few compare or validate these numerous procedures. Without clearly defined roles, the appropriate indications for each remain somewhat arbitrary and subject to further scrutiny. Most of today's surgeons, therefore, are left with choosing what

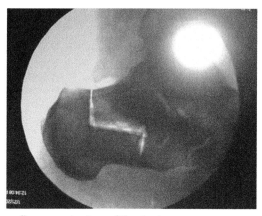

Fig. 3. Postosteotomy fluoroscopic view of Z-osteotomy.

makes sense and what is familiar. In general, though, there are several basic tenets of calcaneal osteotomy that at least enjoy considerable agreement. A posterior displacing osteotomy with superior displacement is likely indicated only when the heel is in calcaneus. These osteotomies are commonly performed in conjunction with plantar fascia release and gastrosoleus recession. Primary heel varus associated with subtle cavus is typically addressed with a lateralizing calcaneal osteotomy. This osteotomy is the least demanding technically, and is reported to have the lowest risk of complication. Complex and severe cavus foot deformities, or revision cases, may require more complex, multiplanar correction. In these cases, consideration of either a Dwyer or the more technically demanding Z-type osteotomies must be given. The Z-osteotomy variants are more challenging to expose, perform, and fix. Although riskier and technically more demanding, a Z-osteotomy also permits greater intraoperative flexibility in dealing with a complex deformity.[3] Because there is no clear algorithm for implementing a calcaneal osteotomy, gaining as much information preoperatively is essential in deciding which osteotomy to implement.

The Coleman block test is critical in understanding the need for a calcaneal osteotomy in treating a cavovarus deformity. The Coleman block test is performed by placing the lateral aspect of the forefoot on a block, allowing the first ray to plantar flex as the heel position is observed (**Fig. 5**).[18] If the heel corrects to a normal valgus, the deformity is deemed flexible and thought to be a forefoot-driven hindfoot varus. This does not require calcaneal osteotomy to derive acceptable correction. If the deformity does not correct, however, the deformity is defined as being fixed or independent of the forefoot (ie, is not forefoot driven). Correction with the Coleman block test suggests a subtler, flexible deformity that can be corrected with a dorsiflexion osteotomy of the first metatarsal and soft tissue balancing. Because adequate correction can be difficult to judge intraoperatively, however, the investigators never rule out performance of a lateralizing calcaneal osteotomy to aid correction when it is thought that additional hindfoot compensation is required.

Radiologic interpretation also contributes to understanding the foot deformity and what level of correction may be required. Weight-bearing ankle and foot views are required preoperatively for all patients. Commonly seen radiologic changes include increased Meary angle, increased calcaneal pitch, increased Hibbs angle, and posteriorly positioned fibula with a flattened talus.[19] Another indication of cavovarus deformity is a vertical-appearing transverse tarsal joint. A lateral radiograph can

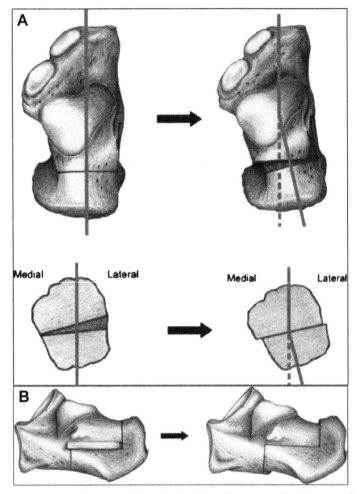

Fig. 4. Z-type osteotomy. (*A*) Illustration showing lateralization and valgisation of the tuberosity after a Z-osteotomy and translation of the calcaneus. (*B*) Illustration showing the site of the osteotomy and the removal of the bone wedge. (*Adapted from* Knupp M, Horisberger M, Hintermann B. A new z-shaped calcaneal osteotomy for 3-plane correction of severe varus deformity of the hindfoot. Tech Foot Ankle Surg 2008;7(2):93; with permission.)

also be taken while the patient is performing a Coleman block test, which indicates the degree of correction obtainable with first metatarsal osteotomy. A computed tomography (CT) scan can further assess not only the hindfoot alignment but also the presence of any dysplasia of the talus or calcaneus that may inhibit reduction of the transverse tarsal joint. However, most CT scans are typically performed non–weight bearing, which can unfortunately misrepresent and confound interpretation of the true clinical alignment under normal conditions.

A Harris axial view can be used to assess hindfoot alignment; however, Saltzman and El-Khoury[7] described specific imaging to assess hindfoot alignment. The hindfoot alignment view provides more information than a calcaneal axial view and better

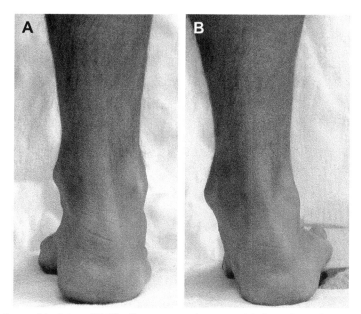

Fig. 5. Coleman block test. (*A*) Hindfoot appears in varus with foot planted on level surface. (*B*) With block under lateral side of forefoot, hindfoot is reassessed. If heel varus corrects, it is suggestive of flexible hindfoot deformity, with secondary heel varus due to valgus forefoot position or plantarflexed first ray.

assessment of hindfoot alignment (**Fig. 6**). Unlike the Harris axial view, the hindfoot alignment view is performed while weight bearing. A specific box is required to obtain the hindfoot alignment and needs to be constructed. Combined with the physical examination, the hindfoot alignment view can give a good idea of the severity of the hindfoot cavus and can be beneficial for selecting which calcaneal osteotomy to perform.

BIOMECHANICS OF CALCANEAL OSTEOTOMY

The effect of a calcaneal osteotomy is often thought of as addressing only the heel varus, but this is perhaps better stated as its primary role. In reality, certain forms of these osteotomies can affect pathology across the entire foot. A thorough understanding of the potential effects of calcaneal osteotomy on the overall foot and ankle alignment is critical. Biomechanical flat foot studies have demonstrated that lateral column lengthening via calcaneal osteotomy alleviates excess forces on the medial arch,[20] while medializing calcaneal osteotomy displaces the calcaneal weight-bearing axis medially. Steffensmeier and colleagues[21] demonstrated an ability to alter the tibio-talar contact zone through both medial and lateralizing calcaneal osteotomy, without globally effecting overall contact pressures. Davitt and colleagues[22] found a minimal effect (less than 10%) on subtalar and tibio-talar contact pressures in a cadaveric model, although these changes were compared with a nonpathologic foot. Krause and colleagues[3] further showed in a cadaveric cavovarus model that all 3 types of common calcaneal osteotomies (Dwyer, lateralizing, and Z-type osteotomies) shifted the hindfoot contact point laterally and improved tibio-talar contact pressures. The Z-shaped osteotomy

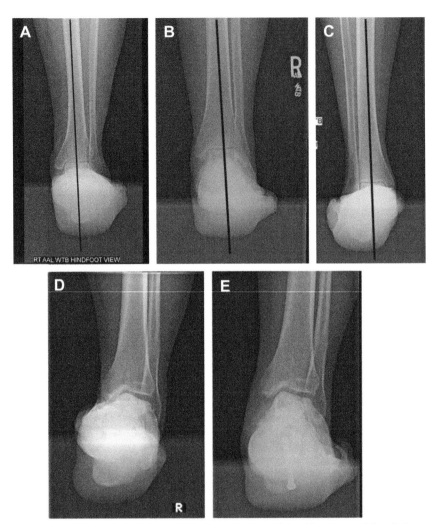

Fig. 6. Example radiographic hindfoot views. (*A*) Normal hindfoot view. (*B*) Subtle varus hindfoot view. (*C*) Valgus hindfoot view. (*D*) Preosteotomy hindfoot view. (*E*) Postosteotomy hindfoot view.

proved to have the greatest effect on shifting the point of contact, whereas lateralizing osteotomy had the greatest impact on tibio-talar contact forces. These differences were not statistically different. Based on our review of the literature, there seems to be consistent alteration of hindfoot biomechanics, but no evidence to support one osteotomy over another in terms of producing a particular biomechanical effect.

CLINICAL RESULTS OF CALCANEAL OSTEOTOMIES

There is a paucity of comparative literature to determine which osteotomy is most appropriate for hindfoot reconstruction in cavovarus deformity. In his series of

170 calcaneal osteotomies for treatment of pes cavus, Dwyer[8] reported 109 of 170 feet demonstrated good to excellent results. Ayres and colleagues[23] reported on 29 Dwyer osteotomies for hindfoot varus with a minimum of 2 years of follow-up that exhibited 89% of patients with good to excellent results. Nayak and Cotterill[24] reported 86% excellent and good results in a series of 42 Dwyer osteotomies in 27 patients with pes cavus with varus heel. Sammarco and Taylor[5] demonstrated 89% good to excellent results in their series of cavovarus foot reconstructions using superiorizing and lateralizing osteotomies, with an average follow-up of 49 months. Maskill and colleagues[25] performed 29 lateral displacement calcaneal osteotomies in combination with metatarsal osteotomies and tendon lengthening and transfers in a series of 23 patients with subtle cavus deformity, and demonstrated a mean improvement from 45 points preoperatively to 90 points postoperatively using the American Orthopaedic Foot and Ankle Society ankle-hindfoot rating system. Knupp and colleagues[14] reported their results on 18 consecutive patients in which a Z-type osteotomy was performed. They showed 17 of 18 patients had good correction in multiple planes without shortening of the calcaneus as may be seen with Dwyer-type osteotomy.

LIMITATIONS OF THE CALCANEAL OSTEOTOMY

Performance of calcaneal osteotomy is certainly not without limitation. The amount of correction obtained is limited by several factors, including osteotomy type, soft tissue constraints, neurovascular compromise, and the osteotomy chosen. The Dwyer osteotomy provides correction in only 1 plane. Significant improvement in heel varus can be seen with a Dwyer osteotomy, but it lacks any translation leading to limited correction and may weaken the Achilles tendon strength.[2] Similarly, the lateralizing calcaneal osteotomy is a single-plane osteotomy that cannot address significant fixed deformities in other planes. Lateralizing calcaneal osteotomies are also limited by the soft tissue surrounding the calcaneus. Krause and colleagues[11] described tarsal tunnel–complicating lateralizing calcaneal osteotomy for cavovarus hindfoot reconstruction in 2 patients with CMT. Ayres and colleagues,[23] in their retrospective study of Dwyer osteotomies, reported 1 patient requiring decompression for tarsal tunnel syndrome. Knupp and colleagues[14] also demonstrated 4 of 18 patients with neurologic examination findings after Z-type osteotomy. Further, we performed a cadaveric study in our laboratory investigating how the magnetic resonance imaging–assessed volume of the tarsal tunnel is affected by calcaneal osteotomy. A statistically significant decrease in tarsal tunnel volume was found associated with lateral shifting of tuber, independent of whether the osteotomy was anteriorly or posteriorly placed.[26] We also identified an important anatomic "safe-zone" relationship related to the location of osteotomy and the neuromuscular structures at risk, as an anterior cut put the neurovascular structures at significantly increased risk of iatrogenic injury as compared with a posterior cut. Based on this work, we now routinely consider a prophylactic tarsal tunnel release when performing a lateralizing calcaneal osteotomy, and advocate strongly for its use in any patients with a stiff soft tissue envelope (rigid contractures), severe primary deformity, or compromised neurophysiology, as seen in patients with CMT disease.

The posterior osteotomy and crescentic osteotomy address only hindfoot cavus. This is a 1-plane osteotomy, there is no valgisation of hindfoot and likely is indicated only in isolated calcaneocavus hindfeet.

Soft tissue contraction on the medial side of the foot can also limit the ability of the surgeon to achieve complete correction. This situation is one of the few times in which medial side incision should be considered.[27] Meticulous techniques are required to prevent soft tissue problems on the medial side and consideration of skin Z-plasty is prudent when severe hindfoot varus is corrected.[27]

In some situations, a calcaneal osteotomy may not provide sufficient correction to completely address the deformity. This is commonly seen in patients in whom the apex of the hindfoot varus is superior to the body of calcaneus.[27] In these situations, the osteotomy is typically combined with subtalar arthrodesis and transverse tarsal osteotomy.

Preoperative arthrosis of the subtalar and/or tibiotalar joints can also limit the ability of a calcaneal osteotomy to achieve desired correction. When these situations are encountered, frequently the calcaneal osteotomy is combined with an arthrodesis procedure or with staged total ankle replacement.

THE AUTHORS' PREFERRED TECHNIQUES
Lateralizing Calcaneal Osteotomy

An oblique incision is made, sufficiently posterior to but parallel with both the peroneal and sural structures, which extend in a posterosuperior to anteroinferior direction over the lateral wall of the calcaneus. This incision is made approximately 1 fingerbreadth below the distal fibula. The subcutaneous tissues are dissected with Bovie electrocautery until the wall of the calcaneus is reached. Care is taken not to undermine the skin and subcutaneous structures in the course of dissection ("canyon walls"). Using a Cobb elevator, the lateral wall of the calcaneus is exposed by blunt elevation of the soft tissues both anteriorly and posteriorly. When the superior and inferior portions of the calcaneal tuber are exposed, Hohman retractors are placed to protect the adjacent dorsal and plantar structures. An oscillating saw is then used to initiate the osteotomy in an oblique fashion, carried through most of the calcaneal tuber parallel to the skin incision and stopping short of penetrating the medial wall. Completion of the osteotomy is carefully performed with the use of an osteotome to gently penetrate the remaining medial cortex of the calcaneus. When completing the inferior portion of the osteotomy, the osteotome and saw are aimed somewhat superior, and vice versa, to reduce the risk of iatrogenic injury to neurovascular structures (**Fig. 7**).

On completion of the cut, a large laminar spreader is placed entirely across the upper half of the osteotomy site to avoid fracture or implosion of the bony surface while distracting the 2 fragments. This also functions to stretch the soft tissues and ease subsequent lateralization. Finally, it permits direct visual inspection of the lower half of the osteotomy and surrounding medial soft tissues. The distractor can then be placed within the inferior region of the calcaneal osteotomy to permit inspection of the dorsal half of the cut. Once the adequacy of the cut is deemed satisfactory for translation and the soft tissues have been inspected, the calcaneal tuber is translated laterally with the use of an elevator and 0.25-inch curved osteotomes follow by dorsiflexion of the foot to compress the osteotomy. The appropriate degree of desired correction (typically 1 cm) is then maintained with 1 or 2 solid 3.2-mm solid drill bits and sequentially stabilized by their replacement with 6.5-mm partially threaded screws with the ankle maintained in neutral dorsiflexion. The subcutaneous tissues are then closed with buried 3-0 Vicryl (Ethicon Endo-Surgery Inc, Cincinnati, OH) sutures and the skin is closed using interrupted 3-0 nylon stitches.

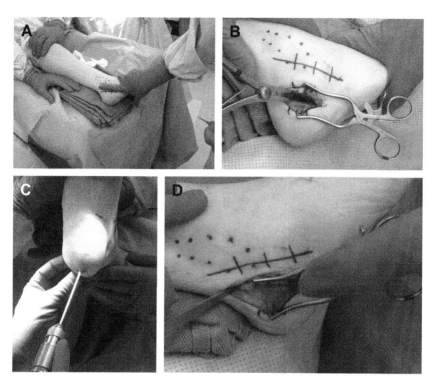

Fig. 7. (*A*) Surgical approach for lateralizing osteotomy is made from the calcaneal tuberosity 1 fingerbreadth behind the fibula. (*B*) An oblique osteotomy is made across the calcaneal tuberosity and opened with a laminar spreader. (*C*) The calcaneal tuberosity is translated and fixation is completed with a 6.5-mm screw predrilled with a 3.2-mm drill bit. (*D*) Correction seen following lateralizing osteotomy.

Triplanar Z-Osteotomy

A Z-osteotomy of the calcaneus is more complex than the standard sliding calcaneal osteotomy and should be approached with even more caution. An oblique incision is made just plantar to the peroneal tendons over the lateral wall of the calcaneus. Care should be taken to avoid injury to the sural nerve, as it can be within the operative field. The lateral wall of the calcaneus is again exposed using blunt dissection with the Cobb elevator. More exposure of the lateral wall of the calcaneus is necessary for the Z-osteotomy, as it requires a larger footprint to complete. Similar to the lateralizing calcaneal osteotomy, the superior and plantar portions of the calcaneus are exposed and Homan retractors are used to visualize the lateral wall of the calcaneus.

Once the exposure is complete, the Z-osteotomy is drawn out on the lateral wall of the calcaneus. The superior limb is typically placed posteriorly and the plantar limb is created anteriorly. The length of the horizontal limb is somewhat dependent on the exposure that is obtained. While protecting the soft tissues, first, the 2 vertical osteotomies are performed. Then the first horizontal limb of the osteotomy is completed, followed by the corrective horizontal limb with size of wedge removed dictated by correction desired. Again, care is taken to complete the osteotomy while not injuring the medial neurovascular tissues (**Fig. 8**).

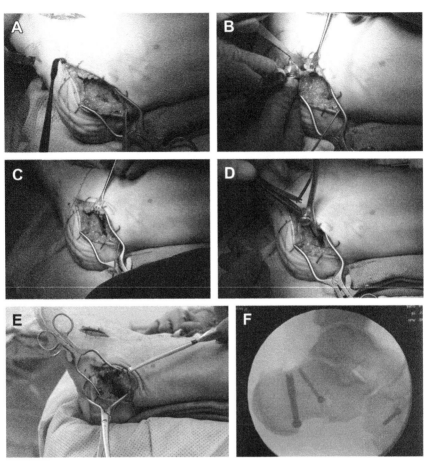

Fig. 8. Operative views of calcaneal Z-osteotomy. (*A*) Horizontal cut for Z-osteotomy. (*B*) Vertical distal cut for Z-osteotomy. (*C*) Z-osteotomy open with Weber clamp. (*D*) Osteotomy site with laminar spreader. (*E*) Osteotomy closed with Weber clamp. (*F*) Postfixation fluoroscopic view.

With the Z-osteotomy completed, wedges of the calcaneus are removed. A horizontal closing wedge is removed from the plantar tuberosity piece to allow for valgisation of the calcaneal tuberosity, while closing vertical wedges are removed from the 2 vertical limbs to allow for external rotation. Once the bony wedges are removed and the osteotomy is distracted with a large laminar spreader, any impeding bony fragments are removed and the calcaneal tuber is reduced. The calcaneal tuber can then undergo lateral translation, valgisation, and external rotation to best correct the deformity. Before stabilization, the correction is visualized using fluoroscopic intraoperative imaging. Once reduced, the osteotomy is stabilized with 1 or 2 partially threaded cannulated screws and again the position is confirmed with intraoperative fluoroscopy. The subcutaneous tissues are closed using buried 3-0 Monocryl (Ethicon Endo-Surgery Inc) suture and the skin is closed using 3-0 nylon suture in an interrupted fashion (**Fig. 9**).

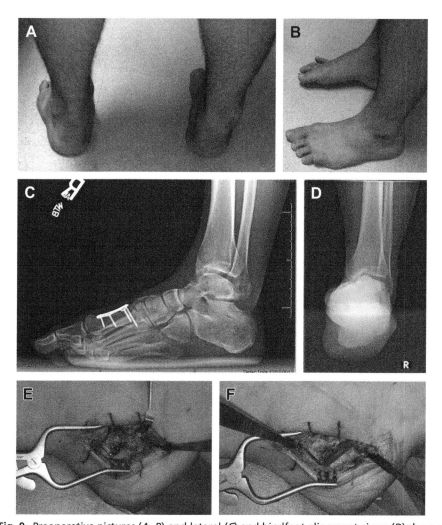

Fig. 9. Preoperative pictures (*A, B*) and lateral (*C*) and hindfoot alignment views (*D*) show a severe hindfoot varus deformity with first-ray dorsiflexion. The patient had a previous Dwyer osteotomy and developed recurrent hindfoot varus thought to be forefoot driven. He subsequently underwent first metatarsal dorsiflexion osteotomy that did not correct his hindfoot varus. Due to failure of the previous Dwyer osteotomy and need for revision surgery, a Z-osteotomy was chosen, as well as a Cotton osteotomy to reverse the first ray dorsiflexion. An oblique lateral incision is made over the tuber of the calcaneus just inferior to the peroneal tendons. The lateral wall of the calcaneus is exposed and a Z-osteotomy is performed with a posterosuperior and anteroinferior vertical limbs connected by a horizontal limb (*E*). Wedges of bone are removed from the horizontal limb and 2 vertical limbs (*F*). The sizes of the bone wedges removed is determined by the amount of correction desired. These wedges allow for valgisation, external rotation, and lateral translation. A laminar spreader is used to displace the osteotomy. The osteotomy is positioned and stabilized with 1 cannulated screw, as seen in the postoperative lateral and hindfoot alignment views (*G, H*). Postoperative clinical pictures show improved hindfoot alignment and forefoot position (*I, J*).

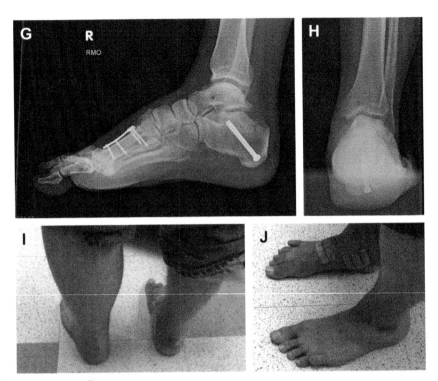

Fig. 9. (*continued*)

SUMMARY

Correction of cavovarus foot deformity is a complex process, and a good surgical outcome requires detailed preoperative assessment of the patient's primary complaint and careful evaluation of the bony and soft tissue characteristics of his or her malalignment. Certainly, calcaneal osteotomy remains a critical cornerstone of management of the cavovarus foot, and many types of these osteotomies have been described. Advantages and disadvantages exist for each, and there is no clear algorithm for when a certain osteotomy should be used. In general, hindfoot varus in a subtle cavovarus foot can be adequately corrected with a lateralizing calcaneal osteotomy with minimal risk. When the hindfoot varus becomes severe or more complex, a Dwyer or Z-calcaneal osteotomy should be strongly considered. However, these osteotomies are inherently more technically difficult and have increased risk associated with them, and therefore should be performed with some basis of familiarity in technique.

REFERENCES

1. Manoli A, Graham B. The subtle cavus foot, "the underpronator". Foot Ankle Int 2005;26(3):256–63.
2. Younger AS, Hansen ST. Adult cavovarus foot. J Am Acad Orthop Surg 2005; 13(5):302–15.
3. Krause FG, Sutter D, Waehnert D, et al. Ankle joint pressure changes in a pes cavovarus model after lateralizing calcaneal osteotomies. Foot Ankle Int 2010; 31(9):741–6.

4. Scranton P, McDermott J, Rogers J. The relationship between chronic ankle instability and variations in mortise anatomy and impingement spurs. Foot Ankle Int 2000;21(8):657–64.

5. Sammarco GJ, Taylor R. Combined calcaneal and metatarsal osteotomies for the treatment of cavus foot. Foot Ankle Clin 2001;6(3):533–43.

6. Dwyer F. Osteotomy of the calcaneum for pes cavus. J Bone Joint Surg Br 1959; 41(1):80–6.

7. Saltzman CL, El-Khoury GY. The hindfoot alignment view. Foot Ankle Int 1995; 16(9):572–6.

8. Dwyer F. The present status of the problem of pes cavus. Clin Orthop Relat Res 1975;(106):254–75.

9. Hansen ST. Osteotomy techniques. In: Functional reconstruction of the foot and ankle. Lippincott Williams & Wilkins; 2000. p. 357–84.

10. Greene DL, Thompson MC, Gesink DS, et al. Anatomic study of the medial neurovascular structures in relation to calcaneal osteotomy. Foot Ankle Int 2001;22(7):569–71.

11. Krause F, Pohl M, Penner M, et al. Tibial nerve palsy associated with lateralizing calcaneal osteotomy: case reviews and technical tip. Foot Ankle Int 2009;30(3): 258–61.

12. Mitchell GP. Posterior displacement osteotomy of the calcaneus. J Bone Joint Surg Br 1977;59(2):233–5.

13. Samilson R, Dillin W. Cavus, cavovarus, and calcaneocavus. An update. Clin Orthop Relat Res 1983;(177):125–32.

14. Knupp M, Horisberger M, Hintermann B. A new z-shaped calcaneal osteotomy for 3-plane correction of severe varus deformity of the hindfoot. Tech Foot Ankle Surg 2008;7(2):90–5.

15. Pisani G. Osteotomia sottotalamica di sottrazione laterale. In: Trattato di chirurgia del piede. Torino (Italy): Edizioni Minerva Medica S.p.A.; 1990. p. 287–8.

16. Malerba F, De Marchi F. Calcaneal osteotomies. Foot Ankle Clin 2005;10(3):523–40.

17. Vermeulen K, Neven E, Vandeputte G, et al. Relationship of the Scarf valgus-inducing osteotomy of the calcaneus to the medial neurovascular structures. Foot Ankle Int 2011;32(5):S540–4.

18. Coleman S, Chesnut W. A simple test for hindfoot flexibility in the cavovarus foot. Clin Orthop Relat Res 1977;(123):60–2.

19. Aminian A, Sangeorzan BJ. The anatomy of cavus foot deformity. Foot Ankle Clin 2008;13(2):191–8.

20. Arangio G, Chopra V, Voloshin A, et al. A biomechanical analysis of the effect of lateral column lengthening calcaneal osteotomy on the flat foot. Clin Biomech 2007;22(4):472–7.

21. Steffensmeier SJ, Saltzman CL, Berbaum KS, et al. Effects of medial and lateral displacement calcaneal osteotomies on tibiotalar joint contact stresses. J Orthop Res 1996;14(6):980–5.

22. Davitt J, Beals T, Bachus K. The effects of medial and lateral displacement calcaneal osteotomies on ankle and subtalar joint pressure distribution. Foot Ankle Int 2001;22(11):885–9.

23. Ayres M, Bakst R, Baskwill D, et al. Dwyer osteotomy: a retrospective study. J Foot Surg 1987;26(4):322–8.

24. Nayak RK, Cotterill C. Dwyer osteotomy in the treatment of pes cavus with varus heel. Foot 1993;3(4):177–83.

25. Maskill M, Maskill J, Pomeroy G. Surgical management and treatment algorithm for the subtle cavovarus foot. Foot Ankle Int 2010;31(12):1057–63.

26. Bariteau J, Bruce B, Sandusky M, et al. Magnetic resonance imaging evaluation of calcaneal ostetomy's effect on tarsal tunnel volume and proximity of nerve structures. Presented at American Academy of Orthopedic Surgeons Annual Meeting. Chicago: 2013.

27. Joseph TN, Myerson MS. Correction of multiplanar hindfoot deformity with osteotomy, arthrodesis, and internal fixation. Instr Course Lect 2005;54:269–76.

Flexible Cavovarus Foot in Children and Adolescents

Kelly L. VanderHave, MD[a],*, Robert N. Hensinger, MD[b],
Brandon W. King, MD[c]

KEYWORDS

- Cavovarus feet • Plantar fascia • Calcaneonavicular ligament
- Calcaneocuboid ligament

KEY POINTS

- Flexible cavovarus feet in children and adolescents can be challenging.
- A careful history and physical examination are paramount for determining the best treatment strategy and a multitude of options are available.
- Specific treatment strategies should be individualized and any bony correction must be in conjunction with a muscle balancing procedure.
- Well-timed soft tissue and occasionally bony procedures can delay the progression of deformity.
- These patients are monitored long term because further treatment may be required.

ANATOMY/BACKGROUND

The arch of foot is unique to *Homo sapiens*, allowing weight distribution and a lever action for upright locomotion. The arch is supported by both osseous and ligamentous structures. The calcaneonavicular (spring) ligament, calcaneocuboid (short plantar) ligament, long plantar ligament, and superficial plantar fascia support the arch.[1]

The medial and central portions of the plantar fascia arise from the calcaneal tuberosity at the medial half of the calcaneus and extend via slips to the transverse metatarsal ligaments that attach to the metatarsal heads. These slips continue distally to the base of the toes on both sides of the flexor tendon sheaths. The plantar fascia stabilizes the arch and prevents the calcaneus from everting, especially when the fascia tightens at push-off. The windlass effect is demonstrated at toe-off, when passive dorsiflexion of

[a] Department of Orthopaedic Surgery, Carolinas Medical Center, 1025 East Morehead, Suite 302, Charlotte, NC 28204, USA; [b] Department of Orthopaedic Surgery, The University of Michigan, 2912 Taubmann Center, Box 0238, 1540 Medical Center Drive, Ann Arbor, MI 48109, USA; [c] Department of Orthopaedic Surgery, The University of Michigan, 2912 Taubman Center, Box 0238, 1500 East Medical Center Drive, Ann Arbor, MI 48109, USA
* Corresponding author.
E-mail address: Kelly.vanderhave@carolinashealthcare.org

Foot Ankle Clin N Am 18 (2013) 715–726
http://dx.doi.org/10.1016/j.fcl.2013.08.006
1083-7515/13/$ – see front matter Published by Elsevier Inc.

the metatarsophalangeal joints places the plantar fascia under tension and elevates the medial arch.[1] Dwyer thought that contracture of the plantar fascia was a principle deforming force in the development of cavus foot deformities.[2]

Pes cavus is a multiplanar foot deformity characterized by an abnormally high medial longitudinal arch. It results from the development of forefoot equinus relative to the position of the hindfoot. The typical cavus foot also has a component of forefoot pronation, which initially involves first metatarsal plantarflexion relative to the hindfoot. The apex of the equinus deformity is usually in the midfoot, most commonly at Chopart joint, but this can be variable.[3,4] Because of the multiple causes and varying severity of cavus foot, the natural history may not be predictable. Cavovarus is defined as plantar flexion of the forefoot with associated hindfoot varus. Conversely, calcaneocavus is defined as forefoot plantar flexion with the hindfoot dorsiflexed.

CAUSE

Population-based studies suggest the prevalence of the cavus foot is approximately 10% to 20%, some of which represent a normal variant.[3,4] An estimated 66% of cavovarus feet are the result of subtle neurologic diseases and conditions that may not become clinically evident until later in life.[5–7] Generally, the cause can be attributed to the brain, spinal cord, peripheral nerves, or muscular/structural problems of the foot. Two-thirds of adults with a symptomatic cavus foot have an underlying neurologic condition, the most common being Charcot-Marie-Tooth (CMT) disease.[5–12] In cases of unknown cause, it can be considered "idiopathic"; however, those labeled idiopathic may likely be the result of a very subtle neurologic lesion below clinical detection.

Peripheral Nerve

CMT is a common cause of cavovarus foot in children and adults but generally is not diagnosed before 10 years of age. Also known as hereditary sensory motor neuropathy (HSMN), it is genetically heterogeneous and usually presents in the first decade of life with delayed motor milestones, distal muscle weakness, clumsiness, and frequent falls. CMT is further classified into subtypes varying in inheritance and progression, as shown in **Table 1**.[13–15] Classification is based on motor nerve conduction velocity studies. Types I, II, and III typically are seen in children. HSMN I, the hypertrophic form of CMT disease, is the most common and has spotty peripheral nerve myelin degeneration and decreased motor nerve conduction. The most common form is HSMN IA, caused by duplication of the gene for peripheral myelin protein 22 (*PMP-22*) on chromosome region 17p11.2. The X-linked form of CMT disease, the second most common form of the disease, is caused by a mutation in the connexin 32 gene. HSMN II, the neuronal form of CMT disease, has an intact myelin sheath with wallerian axonal degeneration, which results in mildly abnormal sensory and motor nerve conduction velocities. HSMN types I and II are both autosomal dominant with variable expression. HSMN III, Dejerine-Sottas disease, is autosomal recessive.[3,4,6,9,11,15–17]

By adulthood, CMT can cause painful foot deformities such as pes cavus. The development of the cavus foot structure seen in CMT has been linked to an imbalance of muscle strength around the foot and ankle (**Table 2**). CMT is characterized by selective anterior and lateral muscle denervation causing muscle imbalance and resultant progressive deformity. The intrinsic muscles atrophy early causing foot shortening and subsequent plantar fascia shortening, which leads to plantarflexion of the first ray with muscle contractions on the hallux creating a forefoot cavus. Hindfoot varus then follows with the plantarflexed first ray causing weight-bearing on the lateral border of the foot.

Table 1
Subtypes of CMT

CMT Type	Inheritance	Features
1	Autosomal-dominant	50% of CMT case Demyelination Slow nerve velocities
1A	—	80% Chromosome 17 PMP-22 defect
1B	—	5%–10% Point mutation of myelin P0 gene Aggressive
1C	—	Unknown
2	Autosomal-dominant	20% Nerve conduction near normal Indolent subtype
X	X-linked	10%–20% Connexin 32 defect Earlier onset More severe
4	Autosomal-recessive	Earlier onset More severe

The new foot position makes the Achilles contribute to further heel inversion and the posterior tibialis tendon is now in a position of mechanical advantage to exacerbate the cavus deformity.[1,2,4,9,13,18,19]

Central Nervous System

Patients with cerebral palsy, particularly hemiplegia, may develop an equinovarus foot due to a spastic tibialis posterior muscle. Occasionally, a calcaneocavus deformity may occur in children with spastic diplegia after an excessively lengthened or released heel cord.[3,4,6] Friedreich ataxia is a familial progressive ataxia in which the posterior column of the spinal cord steadily deteriorates. Children with Friedreich ataxia may first be diagnosed by the occurrence of cavus feet early in the second decade. The full clinical triad includes ataxia, plantar Babinski response, and areflexia. Friedreich ataxia is autosomal recessive and is caused by an abnormal gene on chromosome 9.[5,6] This disorder is often rapidly progressive with no known cures or treatment to

Table 2
Sequence of muscle denervation and force couples in CMT

Muscle Denervation	Force Couple
Intrinsics	Extrinsics > intrinsics
Peroneals (brevis > longus)	Peroneus longus > tibialis anterior
Tibialis anterior	Tibialis posterior > peroneus brevis
Posterior compartment (tibialis posterior, gastrocnemius, soleus)—much later	—

Data from Refs.[11,13,19]

halt progression. Other less common conditions associated with cavovarus feet include Roussy-Levy syndrome and hereditary cerebellar ataxia.[6,11]

Spinal Abnormalities

Static or progressive cavus foot may be associated with developmental spinal abnormalities. Myelodysplasia may cause either unilateral or bilateral cavus foot. Calcaneocavus may be seen in children with diastematomyelia or myelodysplasia, especially when the triceps surae muscle is weak and the tibialis anterior muscle is normal. Syringomyelia or split-cord malformations may be associated with a unilateral cavus foot deformity. Patients with poliomyelitis may present with calcaneocavus. It is distinct from CMT in that the tibialis anterior and intrinsics are usually preserved with paralysis of the gastrocsoleus complex. As a result of paralysis of the triceps surae, the calcaneus is dorsiflexed and the forefoot is plantarflexed. The natural history and management of cavus foot deformities resulting from relatively nonprogressive conditions, such as poliomyelitis, differ substantially from those of cavus foot deformities resulting from progressive diseases.[1,6,9,20] Other causes include spinal cord tumors, intrathecal lipoma, tethered cord syndrome, and Guillain-Barré syndrome. Neurosurgical evaluation and intervention often improve or limit progression of the foot deformity in these circumstances.[5] Peripheral nerve causes include polyneuritis, spinal muscular atrophy, atypical polyneuritis, and neuromuscular choristoma.[5,9,11]

Other Causes

Although the number of neurologic conditions that may lead to cavus foot is extensive, the common factor is muscle imbalance that disrupts the synergy between the intrinsic and extrinsic muscles. Isolated injuries to nerves, muscles, and tendons can result in cavus foot and may provide insight into how specific muscle imbalance can cause a foot deformity. Cavus deformity may occur after an injection injury to the sciatic nerve. The lateral division of the sciatic nerve is more susceptible than the medial division to injury, which may result in weakness of the peroneal and tibialis anterior muscles.[21] Cavus deformity can occur after fibrous contracture of the deep posterior compartment resulting from vascular damage, missed deep compartment syndrome, severe muscle laceration, or a combination of these mechanisms.[1,5] Cavus has been associated with clubfoot or residual clubfoot deformity in 22% of children.[1,22] In clubfoot surgery, placing the navicular in a dorsally subluxated position can lead to postoperative residual cavus foot deformity.[6,23] An understanding of the underlying muscle imbalance in the cavus foot is extremely important for treatment.

CLINICAL PRESENTATION

A strong attempt to determine the cause of cavus foot is important because it may affect prognosis and outcome. Family history (particularly of CMT), birth history, and developmental history are important. Symptoms such as unsteady gait, ankle instability (caused by a combination of weakness and misalignment), pain under the forefoot, or sensory changes in the feet may be present. In addition to foot-related symptoms, hand, hip, foot, and bowel or bladder symptoms should be elicited.[1,6]

PHYSICAL EXAMINATION

A general physical examination should precede a more focused examination of the foot. This more focused examination should include the patient's shoeless gait, spine (sagittal and coronal deformity, midline cutaneous stigmata), and hands (intrinsic atrophy). Unilateral versus bilateral cavus should be established because unilateral involvement suggests an anatomic lesion. CMT disease is likely in the patient with claw toes, cavus foot, poor balance, unsteady gait, and intrinsic hand atrophy. Occasionally, painful hip dysplasia may be the initial presenting problem in a patient with CMT disease. A thorough sensory and motor examination with motor grading should be conducted including deep tendon reflexes to help differentiate upper and lower motor neuron disorders.[1,9,14,18]

Focused examination of the foot should proceed in a systematic way. This examination should include the position of the hindfoot differentiated into cavovarus or calcaneovarus. The apex of the cavus deformity and position of toes should be documented and used for operative planning. A thorough sensory and motor examination with motor grading should be conducted. Specific graded strength of the tibialis anterior, tibialis posterior, and gastrocsoleus complex should be documented.

Calluses suggest decreased flexibility of the foot. Pain from abnormal pressure typically develops at the base of the fifth metatarsal, and first metatarsal head. Toe deformities are common (**Fig. 1**). Abnormal pressures cause the metatarsal fat pad to atrophy and translate distally with time.[1,11,24]

Coleman and Chesnut[25] described the cavovarus test, commonly termed the Coleman block test (**Fig. 2**), to evaluate the pronated forefoot. It assumes that the initial deformity is in the forefoot and is used to determine whether the hindfoot deformity is flexible or fixed. With the heel and lateral border of the foot on a block, the patient is asked to force the first metatarsal head into bearing weight, and the position of the hindfoot is assessed. When the hindfoot is flexible, it remains in neutral and treatment can be limited to the forefoot. This test is done preoperatively to determine if osteotomy of the first ray is needed. In addition, if the hindfoot deformity is rigid, then surgical intervention must address both the forefoot and the hindfoot.[1,3,25,26]

IMAGING
Radiographs

Imaging should start with standing anteroposterior and lateral radiographs of the foot and ankle. Coleman recommended standing anteroposterior and lateral foot radiographs while on the block to document the results of the clinical test. In conditions with forefoot equinus, such as CMT disease, the lateral weight-bearing radiograph shows the calcaneus in neutral dorsiflexion/plantarflexion and the medial forefoot in plantarflexion. In a foot with isolated forefoot equinus, the calcaneus retains its normal relation to the talus. The apex of the deformity can vary. Usually the equinus deformity is located in the midfoot at the transverse tarsal articulation or at the naviculocuneiform joint but does not involve the calcaneus.

Measurement of several radiographic angles is helpful in evaluating the lateral weight-bearing radiograph (**Fig. 3**). On a true lateral view, the lateral and medial

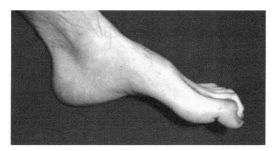

Fig. 1. Claw toes.

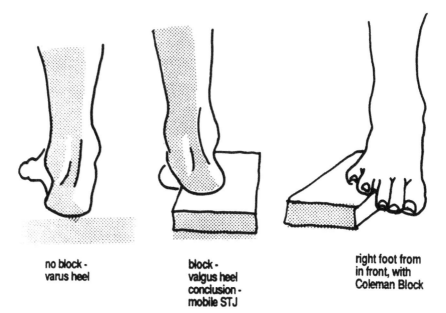

no block -
varus heel

block -
valgus heel
conclusion -
mobile STJ

right foot from
in front, with
Coleman Block

Fig. 2. Coleman block test. (*From* Coleman SS, Chesnut WJ. A simple test for hindfoot flexibility in the cavus foot. Clin Orthop Relat Res 1977;123:61; with permission.)

malleoli will be parallel; however, small differences that are the result of variations in radiographic projection should not influence treatment decisions. Meary's angle is formed by the intersection of 2 lines connecting the long axis of the talus with the long axis of the first metatarsal. It typically measures 0° to 5° in the normal foot but averages 18° in patients with CMT disease. The point of intersection is the apex of the deformity, which is important when considering osteotomies.[1,3,19] Forefoot equinus, or calcaneal pitch, is the angle formed from a line parallel to the floor and a line along the plantar surface of the calcaneus. It is normally about 30° and differentiates

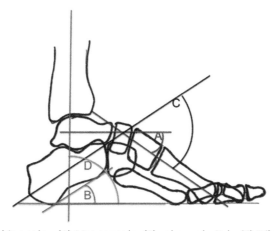

Fig. 3. Radiographic angles: (A) Meary angle; (B) calcaneal pitch; (C) Hibb angle; (D) tibioplantar angle.

a calcaneocavus from a forefoot equinus deformity. A calcaneal pitch less than 30° indicates forefoot equinus rather than calcaneocavus. In calcaneocavus, there is marked dorsiflexion of the calcaneus, a normal medial forefoot, and a calcaneal pitch angle greater than 30°.[1,3,6,19] Hibbs angle is formed by a line through the calcaneus and a line through the axis of the first metatarsal. It is normally less than 45° but can approach 90° in the cavus foot.[1,3,19,27] The weight-bearing tibioplantar angle is measured between the long axis of the tibia and a line from the plantar surface of the calcaneus to the metatarsal heads. It usually measures 90° and is useful when considering a midfoot osteotomy.

If there is clinical evidence for spinal deformity, standing radiographs of the spine should be obtained. In patients with CMT disease, a standing radiograph of the pelvis should be obtained to detect asymptomatic acetabular dysplasia.

Other Diagnostic Evaluation

All patients with unilateral cavus foot deformity should undergo magnetic resonance imaging of the brain and spinal cord to evaluate for anatomic causes including syringomyelia and diastematomyelia. Electrodiagnostic studies can be considered to confirm hereditary motor sensory neuropathies.[12] Because many mutations in different genes have been identified, genetic testing (DNA) is also commonly performed for confirmation of associated neurologic conditions.[1]

MANAGEMENT OF THE FLEXIBLE CAVUS FOOT

To provide the best chance for functional recovery and/or prevent progression in patients with conditions such as a tethered spinal cord, the first step is identification of any treatable underlying cause. The family may need counseling regarding the natural history of the condition, and genetic counseling is mandatory for patients with HSMN. Surgical management may be indicated when functional problems develop or if progressive deformity has been observed. Cavus foot deformity caused by nonprogressive conditions with intact sensation in the foot is more predictable and has a better long-term prognosis. Deformities caused by a tethered spinal cord or lipomeningocele have less predictable outcomes.

NONOPERATIVE MANAGEMENT

Nonoperative management is appropriate for the patient with a mild or nonprogressive deformity. In patients with fixed plantarflexion of the first metatarsal and a flexible hindfoot, a shoe insert that supports the lateral forefoot on posts and thus eliminates the hindfoot inversion may be used. Use of other orthoses depends on the condition and typically consists of unloading areas with excessive pressure and more evenly distributing weight, by use of a metatarsal bar, extra depth shoes, and lateral posts.[5,9,10] Dwyer thought that a bar under the metatarsal heads coupled with passive stretching of the plantar fascia was also effective in controlling dynamic toe deformities. Unloading areas of excessive plantar pressure with foot orthotics and accommodating excessive tarsal or phalangeal height by extradepth shoes may be needed. Patients with weak ankle dorsiflexion may require ankle-foot-orthoses to control footdrop.[6,7,9–16,18,19]

Physical therapy may be useful in adolescents to prevent contractures and preserve proprioception.[3] The injection of botulinum toxin into the peroneus longus and tibialis posterior in CMT patients has not been effective in preventing progression of deformity.[28]

SURGICAL MANAGEMENT OF FLEXIBLE CAVOVARUS FOOT

The goal of surgical management is to obtain a mobile plantigrade foot with correction of the cavus deformity. The type of procedure depends on patient age, level of activity, nature of the deformity, and the cause of the condition. Several principles are central to achieving a satisfactory result. Flexible deformities can be treated with soft tissue procedures. Progressive deformities typically require both soft tissue and bony procedures as well as the use of orthotics after correction. Correction should be obtained at the location of maximum deformity. The underlying muscle imbalance can be corrected by either changing the lever arm that influences the muscle function or by lengthening or transferring the tendons responsible for the deforming forces. A transferred tendon will lose one strength grade; therefore, a muscle should be transferred only when its strength is at least grade 4 when using the tendon transfer for deformity correction.[12] A wide variety of procedures for the treatment of cavovarus foot deformities have been described, but no single combination of procedures has gained wide acceptance.

Toe Deformities

Flexible or passively correctible claw toes may improve spontaneously after correction of the midfoot deformity. Dwyer proposed that postoperative weight-bearing on a better balanced foot would gradually flatten the forefoot and toes.[29] It is advisable to observe patients after correction of the cavus deformity and address toe deformities if still present with a second surgery at a later time. Tendon transfers, such as the Girdlestone-Taylor transfer of the flexor digitorum longus muscle to the extensor hood, can be used for flexible deformities. More fixed deformities require a dorsal metatarsophalangeal capsulotomy or resection arthroplasty. A modified Jones procedure uses a hallucal interphalangeal joint fusion combined with transfer of the extensor hallucis longus tendon to the first metatarsal neck or tarsals (Hibbs technique). This modified Jones procedure removes the deforming force of the extensor hallucis longus tendon on the metatarsophalangeal joint and counteracts the windlass effect on the medial arch by helping to dorsiflex the first metatarsal.[18] Jones transfer to the lesser rays can also be an excellent choice in patients with metatarsalgia secondary to simple pes cavus and long toes. Muller and colleagues[30] noted complete correction of 26 of 33 feet with good to excellent results. Important technical points include avoidance of transfer of more than one extensor tendon to a single metatarsal, sufficiently shortening to prevent clawing, and simultaneous correction of fixed cock-up toes. Care is required as injury to the extensor hallucis brevis can result in a flexion deformity after a modified Jones procedure. Another important technical point is that the peroneus longus is nearly 5 times stronger than the extensor hallucis longus muscle so a transfer of the extensor hallucis longus to the neck of the first metatarsal may not provide sufficient strength to counteract the pull of the peroneus longus.[31]

Soft Tissue Procedures

Cavus foot in patients with progressive conditions requires early, simple procedures. Early soft tissue procedures have been shown to reduce the need for a triple arthrodesis later in life.[15,24] A subcutaneous plantar fascia release may benefit young children with minimal deformity, whereas a complete release including release of the plantar fascia, abductor hallucis, flexor digitorum brevis, quadratus plantae, and abductor digiti quinti muscles is required in more involved cases.[32] This release can be done through a medial- or lateral-based incision, although release of the plantar fascia from the medial side is easier. Postoperative serial casting can be used to slowly correct the cavus deformity. Plantar fascia release also is the initial procedure of choice in young children with nonprogressive deformity. Sherman and Westin reported good success with plantar release through a lateral hindfoot incision for correction of cavus foot in patients with poliomyelitis and clubfoot deformity.[33]

Tendon Transfers

Tendon transfers or lengthenings can be used when there is an identifiable muscle imbalance, especially in younger patients with a flexible deformity. Tendon transfers for muscle rebalancing are also important after osteotomies for preventing recurrence of the deformity after bony correction and can be done within the same surgery, but should be done after osteotomies because the tendon lengths will change. Principles of tendon transfer should be followed, although Myerson and others have stated that even transfers muscles with grade 3 strength will correct deformity and prevent recurrence.[1]

In progressive conditions, transfer of the tibialis posterior tendon through the interosseous membrane to the lateral cuneiform augments dorsiflexion and may prevent varus deformity of the hindfoot.[1,5] In patients with HSMN II, the hindfoot may be in dorsiflexion, and the Achilles tendon should not be lengthened, because this will effectively worsen the calcaneus.[2] Conversely, in equinocavus associated with spastic hemiplegia, the triceps surae muscle may require surgical lengthening in addition to transferring the tibialis posterior, either in whole or as a split transfer to the peroneus brevis tendon. Transfer of peroneus longus to brevis often accompanies a first metatarsal osteotomy.[8] When the deformity is driven by a plantar flexed first ray, as described by Paulos and colleagues, transferring the peroneus longus to the peroneus brevis removes a deforming force on the first ray and reinforces the weak eversion strength of the peroneus brevis.

Forefoot Osteotomies

Patients with fixed forefoot deformity require bony correction of the first ray. A dorsal-based closing-wedge osteotomy of the plantar flexed first metatarsal can be done at the time of the modified Jones procedure. Closing-wedge proximal metatarsal osteotomies require an associated plantar fascia release. In early CMT disease, the functional heel varus is mild and usually corrects after the forefoot osteotomy. Long-term follow-up has shown that this approach uses first metatarsal dorsiflexion osteotomy, peroneus longus to brevis transfer, plantar fascia release, and Jones transfer results in well-maintained correction with a relatively low (20%) rate of reoperation. At an average follow-up of 26.1 years, no patients required triple arthrodesis.[8] Technically, if the first metatarsal is appreciably short, a plantar opening-wedge osteotomy in the skeletally mature foot can be performed. If the major deformity is in the midfoot, correction through the midfoot may provide a better result.

Midfoot Osteotomies

Several types of midfoot osteotomy have been used in children older than 10 years. Midfoot osteotomies require a concomitant plantar fascia release to achieve correction. When done through the first cuneiform bone, correction of the plantar flexed medial column can be achieved at the apex of the deformity. A rocker-bottom deformity and abnormal weight distribution can occur if the osteotomy is performed too distally. Previous studies have shown that only 20° to 25° of tarsometatarsal correction can be obtained in the midfoot.[5]

Several other osteotomies have been described. The Japas V-tarsal osteotomy corrects the deformity at the most prominent point, avoiding the midtarsal joints. It is reportedly simple, results in acceptable shortening, and readily heals.[34] Wilcox and Weiner[35] described the midtarsal dome osteotomy for midfoot cavovarus deformity. The advantages include better control of the forefoot (varus and valgus) as well as plantarflexion/dorsiflexion, while obtaining correction at the apex of the deformity. The authors advocated use of this procedure for children with residual cavus associated with resistant clubfoot deformities and as a salvage procedure in rigid pes cavus. A retrospective review showed satisfactory results in 76% of 106 cases at an average follow-up of 7.6 years with unsatisfactory results being attributed to recurrence.[36–38]

SUMMARY

Flexible cavovarus feet in children and adolescents can be challenging. A careful history and physical examination are paramount for determining the best treatment strategy and a multitude of options are available, which were presented herein. Specific treatment strategies should be individualized and any bony correction must be in conjunction with a muscle-balancing procedure. For progressive conditions, an ankle-foot orthosis is recommended for long-term use even after surgical intervention (**Fig. 4**). Long-term follow-up studies of patients with progressive disease who have had soft tissue procedures and osteotomies are lacking in the literature. The worst prognosis occurs in those patients with early disease onset. Well-timed soft tissue and occasionally bony procedures can delay the progression of deformity. These patients are monitored long term because further treatment may be required.

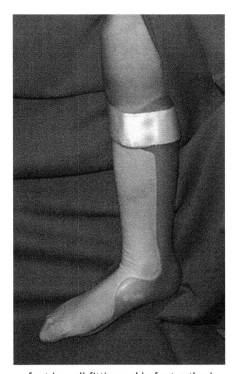

Fig. 4. Bracable cavovarus foot in well fitting ankle foot orthosis.

REFERENCES

1. Lee MC, Sucato DJ. Pediatric issues with cavovarus foot deformities. Foot Ankle Clin 2008;13:199–219.
2. Dwyer FC. Osteotomy of the calcaneus for pes cavus. J Bone Joint Surg Br 1959; 41(1):80–6.
3. Wicart P. Cavus foot, from neonates to adolescents. Orthop Traumatol Surg Res 2012;98(7):813–28.
4. Aminian AA, Sangeorzan BJ. The anatomy of cavus foot deformity. Foot Ankle Clin 2008;13:191–8.
5. Jahss MH. Evaluation of cavus foot for orthopaedic treatment. Clin Orthop Relat Res 1983;181:52–63.
6. Guyton GP. Pes cavus. Coughlin: corrective surgery of the foot and ankle. 8th edition. Philidelphia: Elsevier Mosby; 2007.
7. Brewerton DA, Sandifer PH, Sweetnam DR. Idiopathic pes cavus: an investigation into its aetiology. Br Med J 1963;2:659–61.
8. Ward CM, Dolan LA, Bennett L, et al. Long-term results of reconstruction for treatment of a flexible cavovarus foot in Charcot-Marie-Tooth disease. J Bone Joint Surg Am 2008;90:2631–42.
9. Holmes JR, Hansen ST. Foot fellow's review: foot and ankle manifestations of Charcot-Marie-Tooth disease. Foot Ankle 1993;14(8):476–86.
10. Alexander IJ, Johnson KA. Assessment and management of pes cavus in Charcot-Marie-Tooth disease. Clin Orthop Relat Res 1989;246:273–81.
11. Mann RA, Missirian J. Pathophysiology of Charcot-Marie-Tooth. Clin Orthop Relat Res 1988;234:221–8.
12. Samilson RL, Dillin W. Cavus, cavovarus, and calcaneocavus. Clin Ortho Relat Res 1983;177:125–32.
13. Guyton GP, Mann RA. The pathogenesis and surgical management of foot deformity in Charcot-Marie-Tooth disease. Foot Ankle Clin 2000;5(2):316–26.
14. Beals TC, Nickisch F. Charcot-Marie-Tooth disease and the cavavarus foot. Foot Ankle Clin 2008;13:259–74.
15. Gould N. Surgery in advanced Charcot-Marie-Tooth disease. Foot Ankle 1984; 4(5):267–73.
16. Roper BA, Tibrewal SB. Soft tissue surgery in Charcot-Marie-Tooth disease. J Bone Joint Surg Br 1989;71(1):17–20.
17. Sabir M, Mann RA. Pathogenesis of Charcot-Marie-Tooth disease in coordination with absent or minimal wasting. Clin Orthop Relat Res 1984;184:223.
18. Olney B. Treatment of the cavus foot: deformity in the pediatric patient with Chacot-Marie-Tooth. Foot Ankle Clin 2000;5(2):305–15.
19. Tynan MC, Klenerman L, Helliwell MA, et al. Investigation of muscle imbalance in the leg in symptomatic forefoot pes cavus: a multidisciplinary study. Foot Ankle 1992;13(9):489–501.
20. Banta JV, Sutherland DH, Wyatt M. Anterior tibial transfer to the os calcis with Achilles tenodesis for calcaneal deformity in myelomenigocele. J Pediatr Orthop 1981;1(2):125–30.
21. Guyton GP. Peroneal nerve branching suggests compression palsy in the deformities of Charcot-Marie-Tooth disease. Clin Orthop Relat Res 2006;451: 167–70.
22. Morcuende JA, Dolan LA, Dietz FR, et al. Radical reduction in the rate of extensive corrective surgery for clubfoot using the Pontseti method. Pediatrics 2004;113(2): 376–80.

23. Kremli MK. Fixed forefoot adduction after clubfoot surgery. Saudi Med J 2003; 24(7):742–4.

24. Wukich DK, Maj MC, Bowen JR. A long term study of triple arthrodesis for correction of pes cavovarus in Charcot-Marie-Tooth disease. J Pediatr Orthop 1989; 9(4):433–7.

25. Coleman SS, Chesnut WJ. A simple test for hindfoot flexibility in the cavus foot. Clin Orthop Relat Res 1977;123:60–2.

26. Dahne R. Congenital and acquired neurologic disorders. Chapter 31. Coughlin: corrective surgery of the foot and ankle. 8th edition. Philidelphia: Elsevier Mosby; 2007.

27. Barenfeld PA, Weseley MS, Shea JM. The congenital cavus foot. Clin Orthop Relat Res 1979;79:119–26.

28. Burns J, Scheinberg A, Ryan MM. Randomized trial of botulinum toxin to prevent pes cavus progression in pediatric Charcot-Marie-Tooth disease type 1A. Muscle Nerve 2010;42:262–7.

29. Dwyer FC. The present status of the problem of pes cavus. Clin Orthop Relat Res 1975;106:254–75.

30. Muller T, Dereymaeker G, Fabry G. Jones transfer to the lesser rays in metatarsalgia: technique and long-term follow-up. Foot Ankle Int 1994;15(10):523–30.

31. Silver RL, de la Garza J, Rang M. The myth of muscle imbalance: a study of relative strengths and excursions of normal muscles about the foot and ankle. J Bone Joint Surg Br 1985;67:432–7.

32. McCluskey WP, Lovell WW, Cummings RJ. The cavovarus foot deformity: etiology and management. Clin Orthop Relat Res 1989;247:27–37.

33. Sherman FC, Westin GW. Plantar release in the correction of deformities of the foot in childhood. J Bone Joint Surg Am 1981;63:1382–9.

34. Japas LM. Surgical treatment of pes cavus by tarsal V-osteotomy: preliminary report. J Bone Joint Surg Am 1968;50:927–44.

35. Wilcox PG, Weiner DS. The Akron midtarsal dome osteotomy in the treatment of rigid pes cavus: a preliminary review. J Pediatr Orthop 1985;5:333–8.

36. Weiner DS, Morscher M, Junko JT, et al. The akron dome midfoot osteotomy as a salvage procedure for the treatment of rigid pes cavus. J Pediatr Orthop 2008; 28(1):68–80.

37. Lariviere JY, Miladi L, Dubousset JC, et al. Failure of Dwyer's procedure in internal pes cavus in children. Physiopathological considerations and therapeutic deductions. Rev Chir Orthop 1985;(71):563–73.

38. Wicart P, Seringe R. Plantar opening wedge osteotomy of cuneiform bones combined with selective plantar release and Dwyer osteotomy for pes cavus in children. J Pediatr Orthop 2006;26(1):100–8.

Management of the Rigid Cavus Foot in Children and Adolescents

Dennis S. Weiner, MD[a],*, Kerwyn Jones, MD[b], David Jonah, MA[c],
Martin S. Dicintio, CMT[d]

KEYWORDS

• Rigidity • Cavus • Salvage • Midtarsal • Osteotomy

KEY POINTS

- This article provides a historical review of osteotomies in the management of rigid cavus foot.
- Positives and negatives of the various historical osteotomies are outlined.
- Akron dome midfoot osteotomy is performed at the apex of deformity.
- Akron dome midfoot osteotomy is capable of complete multidirectional correction of deformity.

Although the complexity of the rigid cavus foot has been appreciated for roughly 100 years, a myriad of surgical options have failed to yield consensus on the appropriate treatment selection applicable to the rigid cavus foot for any given origin.

Nearly a century has passed since Arthur Steindler[1–3] in 1917, 1920, and 1921 published a series of articles relative to the structure and management of the complex and rigid cavus foot. In addition to the procedure involving "stripping of the plantar fascia," which bears his name, he proposed a dorsal-based wedge osteotomy through the neck of the talus, including the distal promontory of the os calcis and proximal cuboid. A plethora of articles addressing the rigid cavus foot have been published since Foley[4] in 1924, Saunders[5] in 1935, Cole[6] in 1940, and Brockway[7] in 1940 presented their approach espousing a dorsal-based wedge through the midfoot. All of these procedures and myriad of others provided uniplanar or biplanar correction at best, until Japas[8] in 1968 reported on a dorsal-based V-wedge osteotomy that provided for a

No direct or indirect commercial financial incentive was associated with this publication. The authors declare no conflict of interest.

[a] Department of Pediatric Orthopaedic Surgery, Children's Hospital Medical Center of Akron, 300 Locust Street, Suite 160, Akron, OH 44302, USA; [b] Department of Pediatric Orthopaedic Surgery, Children's Hospital Medical Center of Akron, Considine Professional Building, 215 West Bowery Street, Suite 7200, Akron, OH 44308, USA; [c] Medical Illustrator, 1211 Oreganum Court, Belcamp, MD 21017, USA; [d] Department of Pediatric Orthopaedic Surgery, Children's Hospital Medical Center of Akron, 300 Locust Street, Suite 250, Akron, OH 44302, USA
* Corresponding author.
E-mail address: dweiner@chmca.org

Foot Ankle Clin N Am 18 (2013) 727–741
http://dx.doi.org/10.1016/j.fcl.2013.08.007
foot.theclinics.com

multiplanar correction. Rotational correction was somewhat restricted in the Japas procedure because of the impinging limbs of the V-osteotomy, but dorsiflexion/plantar flexion and varus/valgus rotation could readily be obtained. Many of the uniplanar or biplanar approaches are discussed in this article, including metatarsal osteotomies, midfoot osteotomies, osteotomies with external fixation, and combined opening medial and closing lateral approaches.

In 1985, Wilcox and Weiner[9] initially proposed the Akron dome midfoot osteotomy. In 1994, Weiner and Weiner[10] reviewed a large series of cases, and Weiner and colleagues[11] in 2008 again described the results in 89 patients with 139 feet, all performed by a single surgeon (D.S.W.). The osteotomy is centered at the apex of the cavus deformity in the frontal, lateral, and plantar planes at the confluence of the longitudinal and transverse arches of the foot. The apex of the deformities is nearly always based at the medial cuneiform bone. Multiplanar correction can be fully obtained, including dorsal plantar, varus-valgus, and rotation in all planes, above and beyond any of the previously reported procedures.

Common causes seen in the early to mid-20th century included, most commonly, infantile paralysis (polio); other neurologic disorders, including cerebral palsy and Charcot-Marie-Tooth disease; and some congenital deformities, such as idiopathic clubfoot. In the 2008 publication by Weiner and colleagues,[11] idiopathic clubfoot was seen most commonly, likely as a consequence of the profound positive effect of the polio vaccine. Other neurologic disorders were the next most prevalent, as they were a century ago. The surgical details of the Akron dome midfoot osteotomy are presented later in this article.

It is an illusion to conceive of any operative procedure restoring these feet to normality. All reported operative procedures to date are salvage by design. The inherent structural rigidity of the midtarsal joints preclude consideration of using joint-sparing approaches. Healing of all of these osteotomies results in arthrodesis, fibrodesis, or simple bony union, ideally with varying degrees of deformity correction.

METATARSAL OSTEOTOMIES

A substantial number of metatarsal osteotomies designed for correction of the rigid cavus have been described throughout the literature.[12–25] The disadvantage of performing the correction at this level is that, although it provides for correction in the forefoot, the apex of the deformity lies within the midfoot region. In nearly all cases, the apex of the rigid cavus is located at the level of the medial cuneiform.[9–11,26] Correction of the cavus deformity with metatarsal osteotomies is often combined with plantar fascia release to allow further cavus correction.

Gould[13] suggested dorsal closing-wedge incomplete (greenstick) osteotomies at the bases of the metatarsals. These greenstick osteotomies maintain rotational alignment. Sammarco and Taylor[23] recommended selective osteotomies of the metatarsals through one dorsal incision for the first and second rays, and continuing with a second dorsal incision if needed to address additional rays. Steytler and Van der Walt[18] recommended a V-shaped osteotomy of the metatarsus with the apex pointing toward the heel to obtain more optimal correction of the frontal plane deformity.

Jahss[17] in 1980 (**Fig. 1**) described a procedure that used a single incision and truncated dorsal wedge osteotomies of the tarsometatarsal joints. The procedure involved excision of bone mostly from the bases of the second and third metatarsals than from the first, fourth, and fifth metatarsal bases. This metatarsal-tarsal joint osteotomy allowed for more dorsoplantar correction. The procedure, although slightly proximal to the other metatarsal osteotomies, still commonly resulted in a dorsal bony

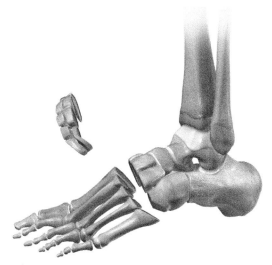

Fig. 1. Lateral view of Jahss osteotomy.

prominence of the midtarsus. Although all of these metatarsal osteotomies lie distal to the apex of the cavus deformity, they leave a residual dorsal bony prominence ("hump") proximally.

PROXIMAL MIDTARSAL AND MIDFOOT BIPLANAR OSTEOTOMIES

Surgical correction of the rigid cavus deformity dates back to Steindler,[1–3] who reported on an approach to the rigid cavus foot via a dorsal-based wedge osteotomy through the talar neck passing plantar-wise through the distal promontory of the calcaneus and the proximal cuboid (**Fig. 2**). This osteotomy was typically combined

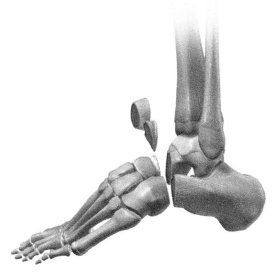

Fig. 2. Lateral view of Steindler osteotomy.

with a plantar stripping (recession of the plantar fascia and short flexors) to diminish their bowstring effect on the cavus, and Steindler subsequently received eponymous recognition of the procedure. The plantar surgical release was facilitated by dorsiflexing the foot and toes at the time of release.

Subsequently, Foley[4] in 1924, Saunders[5] in 1935, and Cole[6] in 1940 (**Fig. 3**) described an osteotomy for cavus deformity dorsally based through the navicular and the medial cuneiform combined with a wedge cuboid osteotomy. The wedge of bone removed was based dorsally, and the apex plantar. The axis of this osteotomy was at the junction of the frontal and sagittal planes, and therefore maximized sagittal plane correction. One concern with this osteotomy is that the forefoot adductus can be increased because of a larger portion of bone being removed medially than the portion removed laterally. Modifying this osteotomy from the dorsomedial to the plantar lateral axis allows for a more appropriate correction of the adductus portion of the deformity.[27] This procedure was performed through 2 incisions (medial and lateral), allowing for deep dissection of the tissue planes to connect each other. A plantar-based wedge of bone is removed from the cuneiforms and navicular. A plantar flexion closing osteotomy of the cuboid is performed through the lateral incision, and the foot is dorsiflexed into a corrected position. The Steindler, Saunders, and Cole osteotomies provide biplanar correction of the cavus deformity but insufficient rotational correction.

An abundance of other similar modifications of midfoot biplanar osteotomy have been described over the years,[28–37] with similar degrees of correction and similar limitations in the degree of multiplanar correction.

MEDIAL-LATERAL MIDFOOT BIPLANAR OSTEOTOMIES

When viewed in the frontal plate, the midfoot and forefoot region can be perceived as consisting of medial and lateral columns. These 2 columns can be architecturally balanced to provide biplanar correction. Various combinations of medial opening and lateral closing wedge osteotomies have been described in this regard (**Fig. 4**).

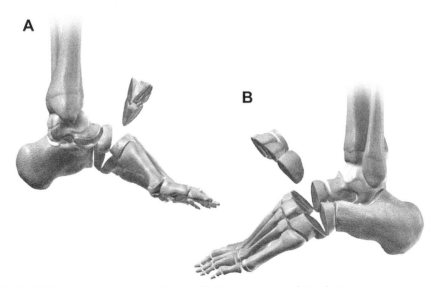

Fig. 3. (*A*) Cole osteotomy, medial view. (*B*) Cole osteotomy, lateral view.

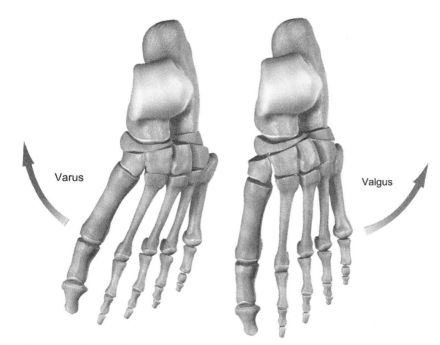

Varus

Valgus

Fig. 4. Frontal view, medial opening and lateral closing wedge osteotomies.

Redirecting the wedges in a slightly plantar or dorsal direction may provide additional correction of midfoot cavus. Adopting this combined approach has led to several similar surgical techniques that provide biplanar correction with minimal disruption of the midfoot joints (joint sparing). One must remember that these joints are inherently rigid (stiff).

In 1991, McHale and Lenhart[38] described a bicolumn osteotomy for the residual clubfoot deformity that they termed the *bean-shaped foot*. Two incisions, one laterally based and one medially based, are used to address the 2 columns of the foot. The lateral column is effectively shortened using a laterally closing wedge osteotomy in the cuboid. Through the medial incision, after protecting the anterior tibialis tendon insertion, an opening wedge osteotomy is created through the medial cuneiform. The wedge-shaped section of bone from the cuboid can be transferred to the opening wedge in the medial cuneiform. Cadaver dissections revealed that the midfoot alterations occurred via closing wedge osteotomy of both the cuboid and medial cuneiform. Other authors[39–42] have reported satisfactory results using this type of surgical approach.

Several authors have described a similar bicolumn procedure, with slight modifications to include an additional transverse osteotomy through the remaining cuneiforms[39,42–47] and small, wedge-shaped osteotomies performed through the remaining cuneiforms.[47] Harley and colleagues,[44] Mahadev and colleagues,[48] and Brink and Levitsky[47] developed bicolumn osteotomies with a wedge removed from the cuboid and a straight transverse osteotomy through the remaining cuneiforms.

These procedures have the advantage of providing satisfactory biplanar correction, but they are likewise limited in rotational correction.

MULTIPLANAR CORRECTION WITH EXTERNAL FIXATION

Several small pin external fixators have been used to correct residual rigid cavus deformities. These adaptable devices offer a distinct advantage for deformity correction of all types because of their ability to achieve correction in multiple planes. The use of these fixators has been described in numerous small case series. Several methods have been used to correct the deformities through distraction histogenesis without osteotomy[49–59] and distraction with osteotomies.[60–63] Typically, extension of the external fixator system above the ankle is supported by most surgeons.

Two commonly used osteotomies are the U-shaped and V-shaped osteotomies. The U-shaped osteotomy is a semicircular osteotomy of the talus. It begins in the posterior and superior body of the talus and extends anteriorly through the talar neck. The V-shaped osteotomy is directed through the calcaneus and talus. The posterior limb of this osteotomy begins in the superior portion of the calcaneal tuberosity and continues in a plantar direction, with the apex of the osteotomy at the mid-planar region of the calcaneus. The anterior portion then continues superiorly, traversing through the neck of the talus. U-shaped osteotomies are intended to correct the entire foot relative to the leg, whereas the V-shaped osteotomy is intended to provide individual correction of the hindfoot, midfoot, and forefoot.[58] Distraction osteotomies can provide satisfactory correction for feet with significant stiffness, including feet with prior fusions.

Distraction histogenesis is another technique used that avoids osteotomies or any other surgical procedure on the foot, except for the percutaneous placement of pins. It offers the advantage of permitting weight-bearing on the limb soon after surgery. Additional advantages of distraction histogenesis include the fact that the surgery, as described by Ilizarov,[64] is essentially bloodless. In addition, correction can be multiplanar and occurs through the joints themselves, providing correction at the site of deformity. Disadvantages include a fairly high recurrence rate and postoperative stiffness in the foot. Grill and Franke[57] reported postoperative stiffness of the subtalar and midtarsal joints. Other disadvantages include those common to all external fixators, including increased risk of pin tract infection, loss of correction, stiffness, increased recurrence rates, and design and application complexity.

MULTIPLANAR OSTEOTOMIES

The deformity in a rigid cavus foot is typically a multiplanar 3-dimensional rigid bone deformity. Japas[8] in 1968 described the first extensive multiplanar V-shaped osteotomy of the tarsals that provided correction in all planes (**Fig. 5**). The osteotomy is approached through a longitudinal dorsal incision. A second, small medial incision is used for a plantar fascia release. The apex of the osteotomy is centered dorsally at the apex of the deformity and has 2 limbs. One extends distally and medially to exit the medial border of the foot at the medial cuneiform, and the second is laterally based, extending distally to exit the lateral border of the foot at the mid cuboid. A skid is used to lever the distal portion of the osteotomy so that the distal end is raised and the proximal end is plantar flexed. Abduction or adduction can be corrected through manipulating the forefoot without removing or adding any bone. Dorsal-plantar and varus-valgus correction can be readily achieved. Moderate rotational correction can be achieved but is limited by abutment of the V-shaped osteotomy limbs. The major advantage of this procedure lies in its ability to correct deformities in all planes, although rotation is limited.

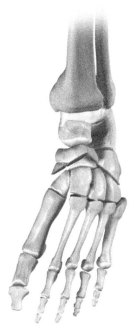

Fig. 5. Superior view of Japas' V-shaped osteotomy.

AKRON DOME MIDFOOT OSTEOTOMY

The Akron dome midfoot osteotomy was designed to correct all types of cavus defor-mities regardless of origin (**Fig. 6**).[9–11] The indications for the procedure were any cavus deformity with less than 50% of the foot plantigrade (subjective observation) with or without symptomatic abnormal weight-bearing pressure areas. The goal of sur-gical treatment is to obtain a plantigrade painless foot. It was never anticipated in any regard that existing hindfoot deformities (equinus, varus or valgus, or deformity distal to the metatarsal necks) would be affected by this procedure in either a positive or a negative fashion.

The surgical technique is initiated by a transverse incision over the dorsum of the foot at the level of the midfoot that is consistently centered at the apex of the deformity at the confluence of the transverse and longitudinal arches. Multiple vertical and soft tissue windows are created down to the capsules of the midfoot joints while avoiding and protecting the neurovascular bundle and extensor tendons. A curved osteotomy is then used to fashion 2 roughly parallel dome-shaped osteotomy cuts across the midfoot, wider dorsally than plantar to allow for rotation of the forefoot out of the equi-nus position, and thereby lowering the longitudinal arch (at the apex of deformity) (**Fig. 7**). Appropriate wedging of the osteotomy cuts is then used to accommodate any directional alteration for varus, valgus (**Fig. 8**), dorsiflexion, plantar flexion (**Fig. 9**), or rotation. A rongeur or power burr is used to facilitate the fine contouring of the opposing osteotomized fragments. In the lateral view, the distal midtarsus and forefoot are rotated out of equinus and the cavus is reduced to a desired position. Varus or valgus is simultaneously corrected through rotating and abducting or adduct-ing the distal component of the osteotomy into the desired position (multidirectional). Once adequate correction is achieved, the foot is maintained in position by 2 crossed

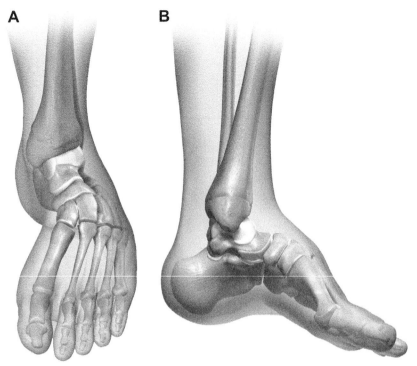

Fig. 6. (A) Frontal view of typical rigid cavovarus foot. (B) Lateral view of typical rigid cavovarus foot.

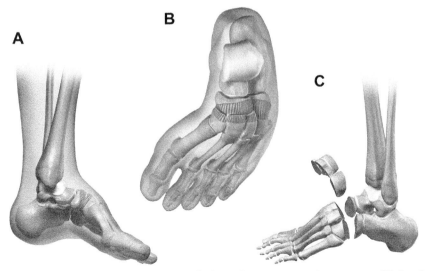

Fig. 7. (A) Surgical oblique lateral view of Akron dome metatarsal osteotomy. (B) Surgical oblique frontal view of Akron dome metatarsal osteotomy. (C) Wedge resection lateral view of Akron dome metatarsal osteotomy.

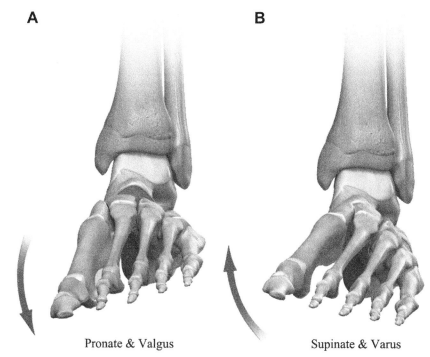

A

B

Pronate & Valgus   Supinate & Varus

Fig. 8. (*A*) Frontal view of Akron dome metatarsal osteotomy showing pronation and valgus. (*B*) Varus-valgus view of Akron dome metatarsal osteotomy showing supination and varus.

percutaneous pins and directed from the medial side of the base of the first metatarsal proximally and directed posterolaterally at a 45° angle, with the second pin being inserted percutaneously at the base of the fifth metatarsal on the plantar side and directed posteromedially at roughly a 45° angle across the osteotomy site (**Fig. 10**). A fine power burr is used to contour any irregularities of the dorsal surfaces at the site of the osteotomy. The skin is closed with an absorbable running suture in a sub-cuticular fashion. A short leg, well-padded cast is applied at completion of the proce-dure. The short leg cast is left in place for 6 weeks, after which the cast and pins are removed in an office setting. A new short leg walking cast is applied for an additional 4 weeks. A plastic ankle/foot orthosis is worn until the fusion is clinically and radio-graphically solid (usually 3–4 months from the date of surgery) (**Figs. 11** and **12**).

DISCUSSION

One must keep in mind that all of these operations are primarily salvage surgeries performed in complex cases with fixed bony rigidity. The Akron dome osteotomy ad-dresses the center of the deformity and provides full multidirectional correction. At the conclusion of the operative procedure, the versatility of the procedure allows for the distal foot to be rotated or manipulated into any desirable position of correction. In 2008, the authors reported that failures of the procedure seemed to be related to the following issues:

- The age of the patient. Younger patients were more likely to experience recur-rence of deformity with continued growth (satisfactory results were 82% for

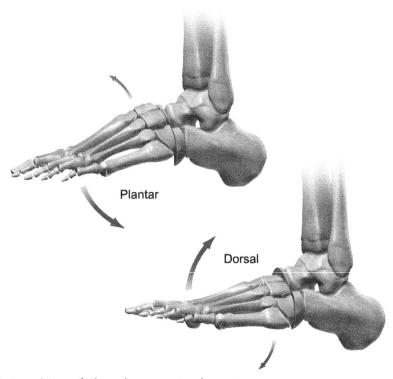

Fig. 9. Lateral view of Akron dome metatarsal osteotomy.

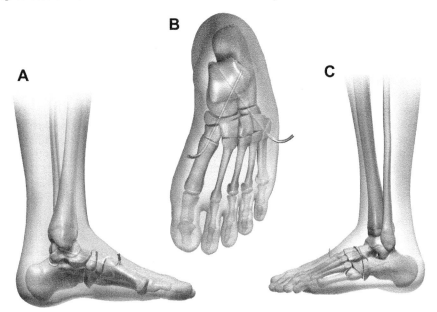

Fig. 10. (*A*) Lateral view of Akron dome metatarsal osteotomy with pin fixation. (*B*) Superior view of Akron dome metatarsal osteotomy. (*C*) Medial view of Akron dome metatarsal osteotomy with pin fixation.

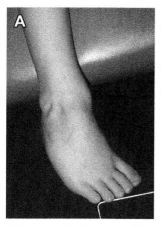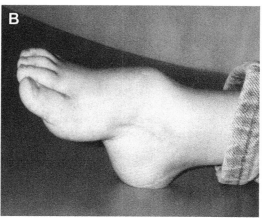

Fig. 11. Example of preoperative patient with a typical clinical cavus deformity. (*A*) Frontal view. (*B*) Side view. (*From* Weiner DS, Morscher M, Junko JT, et al. The Akron dome midfoot osteotomy as a salvage procedure for the treatment of rigid pes cavus: a retrospective review. J Pediatr Orthop 2008;28(1):70; with permission.)

$\geq$8 years of age vs 67% for <8 years of age). However, some of the patients younger than 8 years had sufficiently severe deformities, such as pain or impending pressure ulcers, that led to earlier surgery than was desired.

- The severity of the initial deformity. Increased severity correlated with inability to obtain satisfactory early correction, resulting in rigid cavus deformity and a need for midfoot osteotomy at an earlier age than was desired.
- Neuromuscular disease that may involve progressive muscle weakness and subsequent deformity.
- The presence of coexisting distal forefoot or hindfoot deformities requiring additional surgery to address those deformities (eg, osteotomies of neck or

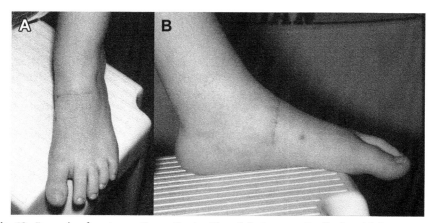

Fig. 12. Example of postoperative patient with satisfactory result—final multiplanar correction. (*A*) Frontal view. (*B*) Side view. (*From* Weiner DS, Morscher M, Junko JT, et al. The Akron dome midfoot osteotomy as a salvage procedure for the treatment of rigid pes cavus: a retrospective review. J Pediatr Orthop 2008;28(1):69; with permission.)

metatarsals, triple or subtalar osteotomy, calcaneal osteotomies). The authors concluded that the optimal patient was older than 8 years without a progressive neurologic disorder, regardless of other origins for the coexisting deformities.

The reported complications of the Akron dome midfoot osteotomy included superficial skin slough and cellulitis, all resolving in time.[11] No cases of deep infection or neural injury were encountered. No perceived shortening occurred, presumably as a result of rotating the forefoot out of equinus and obtaining a more plantigrade position of the foot (relative lengthening). The architectural changes in achieving a plantigrade position seem to compensate for most of the bone removal (limiting potential shortening) at the site of osteotomy.

Deformity in the hindfoot or distal to the neck of the metatarsals will not likely be affected by any midtarsal osteotomy. Nonetheless, substantial correction of the rigid cavus deformity can be expected, particularly if multiplanar correction can be achieved.

SUMMARY

In light of the historical evaluation of surgical approaches to the rigid cavus feet, attempts at extensive multiplanar corrections centered at the apex of the deformity seem to have provided the best options for maximum correction.

Although a multitude of surgical options exist for the management of rigid cavus deformity in children and adolescents, the Akron dome midfoot osteotomy seems to offer the best current option for multiplanar correction, regardless of origin.

REFERENCES

1. Steindler A. Operative treatment of pes cavus. Surg Gynecol Obstet 1917;24:612–5.
2. Steindler A. Stripping of the os calcis. J Bone Joint Surg Am 1920;2:8–12.
3. Steindler A. The treatment of pes cavus (hollow claw foot). Arch Surg 1921;2:325–7.
4. Foley TM. Pes cavus, due to paralysis of the extensor muscles, dorsal flexors of the feet. South Med J 1924;17:798–800.
5. Saunders JT. Etiology and treatment of clawfoot: report of the results in one hundred and two feet treated by anterior tarsal resection. Arch Surg 1935;30:179–98.
6. Cole WH. The treatment of claw-foot. J Bone Joint Surg Am 1940;22:895–908.
7. Brockway A. Surgical correction of cavus deformities. J Bone Joint Surg Am 1940;22:81–9.
8. Japas LM. Surgical treatment of pes cavus by tarsal V-osteotomy. Preliminary report. J Bone Joint Surg Am 1968;50:927–44.
9. Wilcox PG, Weiner DS. The Akron midtarsal dome osteotomy in the treatment of rigid pes cavus: a preliminary review. J Pediatr Orthop 1985;5:333–8.
10. Weiner BK, Weiner DS. The Akron midtarsal dome osteotomy in the treatment of rigid pes cavus. In: Simons GW, editor. Clubfoot. New York: Springer-Verlag; 1994. p. 377–83.
11. Weiner DS, Morscher M, Junko JT, et al. The Akron dome midfoot osteotomy as a salvage procedure for the treatment of rigid pes cavus: a retrospective review. J Pediatr Orthop 2008;28:68–80.
12. Swanson AB, Braune HS, Coleman JA. The cavus foot concept of production and treatment by metatarsal osteotomy. J Bone Joint Surg Am 1966;48:1019.

13. Gould N. Surgery in advanced Charcot-Marie-Tooth disease. Foot Ankle 1984;4: 267–73.
14. Alvik I. Operative treatment of pes cavus. Acta Orthop Scand 1953;23: 137–41.
15. Alexander IJ, Johnson KA. Assessment and management of pes cavus in Charcot-Marie-tooth disease. Clin Orthop Relat Res 1989;246:273–81.
16. Jahss MH. Evaluation of the cavus foot for orthopedic treatment. Clin Orthop Relat Res 1983;181:52–63.
17. Jahss MH. Tarsometatarsal truncated-wedge arthrodesis for pes cavus and equinovarus deformity of the fore part of the foot. J Bone Joint Surg Am 1980; 62:713–22.
18. Steytler JC, Van der Walt ID. Correction of resistant adduction of the forefoot in congenital club-foot and congenital metatarsus varus by metatarsal osteotomy. Br J Surg 1966;53:558–60.
19. Wang GJ, Shaffer LW. Osteotomy of the metatarsals for pes cavus. South Med J 1977;70:77–9.
20. McElvenny RT, Caldwell GD. A new operation for correction of cavus foot; fusion of first metatarsocuneiformnavicular joints. Clin Orthop 1958;11:85–92.
21. Gudas CJ. Mechanism and reconstruction of pes cavus. J Foot Surg 1977;16: 1–8.
22. Watanabe RS. Metatarsal osteotomy for the cavus foot. Clin Orthop Relat Res 1990;252:217–30.
23. Sammarco GJ, Taylor R. Cavovarus foot treated with combined calcaneus and metatarsal osteotomies. Foot Ankle Int 2001;22:19–30.
24. Dwyer FC. The present status of the problem of pes cavus. Clin Orthop Relat Res 1975;106:254–75.
25. Johnson JB. A preliminary report on chondrotomies: a new surgical approach to metatarsus adductus in children. J Am Podiatry Assoc 1978;68:808–13.
26. Mosca VS. The foot. In: Morrissy RT, Weinstein SL, editors. Lovell and Winter's pediatric orthopaedics. 5th edition. Philadelphia: Lippincott Williams & Wilkins; 2001. p. 1151–215.
27. Harley BD. Cole midfoot osteotomy. In: Lasday SD, Pachuda NM, Jay RM, editors. Pediatric foot and ankle surgery. Philadelphia: WB Saunders; 1999. p. 220–4.
28. McCluskey WP, Lovell WW, Cummings RJ. The cavovarus foot deformity. Etiology and management. Clin Orthop Relat Res 1989;247:27–37.
29. Leal LO, Bosta SD, Feller DP. Anterior tarsal resection (Cole osteotomy). J Foot Surg 1988;27:259–63.
30. Levitt RL, Canale ST, Cooke AJ Jr, et al. The role of foot surgery in progressive neuromuscular disorders in children. J Bone Joint Surg Am 1973;55: 1396–410.
31. Johnson BM, Child B, Hix J, et al. Cavus foot reconstruction in 3 patients with Charcot-Marie-Tooth disease. J Foot Ankle Surg 2009;48:116–24.
32. Shapiro F, Bresnan MJ. Orthopaedic management of childhood neuromuscular disease. Part II: peripheral neuropathies, Friedreich's ataxia, and arthrogryposis multiplex congenita. J Bone Joint Surg Am 1982;64:949–53.
33. Wülker N, Hurschler C. Cavus foot correction in adults by dorsal closing wedge osteotomy. Foot Ankle Int 2002;23:344–7.
34. Groner TW, DiDomenico LA. Midfoot osteotomies for the cavus foot. Clin Podiatr Med Surg 2005;22:247–64.
35. Stapleton JJ, DiDomenico LA, Zgonis T. Corrective midfoot osteotomies. Clin Podiatr Med Surg 2008;25:681–90.

36. Tullis BL, Mendicino RW, Catanzariti AR, et al. The Cole midfoot osteotomy: a retrospective review of 11 procedures in 8 patients. J Foot Ankle Surg 2004; 43:160–5.

37. Erotas JT, Beal WS. Cuneiform wedge osteotomy: a new approach to the correction of a rigid plantargrade medial column. J Foot Surg 1986;25:364–8.

38. McHale KA, Lenhart MK. Treatment of residual clubfoot deformity—the "bean-shaped" foot—by opening wedge medial cuneiform osteotomy and closing wedge cuboid osteotomy. Clinical review and cadaver correlations. J Pediatr Orthop 1991;11:374–81.

39. Schaefer D, Hefti F. Combined cuboid/cuneiform osteotomy for correction of residual adductus deformity in idiopathic and secondary club feet. J Bone Joint Surg Br 2000;82:881–4.

40. Loza ME, Bishay SN, El-Barbary HM, et al. Double column osteotomy for correction of residual adduction deformity in idiopathic clubfoot. Ann R Coll Surg Engl 2010;92:673–9.

41. Dehne R. Osteotomy in the pediatric foot. Foot Ankle Clin 2001;6:599–614.

42. Lourenco AF, Dias LS, Zoellick DM, et al. Treatment of residual adduction deformity in clubfoot: the double osteotomy. J Pediatr Orthop 2001;21:713–8.

43. Köse N, Günal I, Göktürk E, et al. Treatment of severe residual clubfoot deformity by trans-midtarsal osteotomy. J Pediatr Orthop B 1999;8:251–6.

44. Harley BD, Fritzhand AJ, Little JM, et al. Abductory midfoot osteotomy procedure for metatarsus adductus. J Foot Ankle Surg 1995;342:153–62.

45. Paulos L, Coleman SS, Samuelson KM. Pes cavovarus. Review of a surgical approach using selective soft-tissue procedures. J Bone Joint Surg Am 1980; 62:942–53.

46. Anderson DJ. Combined lateral column shortening and medial column lengthening in the treatment of severe forefoot adductus. Orthop Trans 1991;15:768.

47. Brink DS, Levitsky DR. Cuneiform and cuboid wedge osteotomies for correction of residual metatarsus adductus: a surgical review. J Foot Ankle Surg 1995;34: 371–8.

48. Mahadev A, Munajat I, Mansor A, et al. Combined lateral and transcuneiform without medial osteotomy for residual clubfoot for children. Clin Orthop Relat Res 2009;467:1319–25.

49. Ferreira RC, Costo MT, Frizzo GG, et al. Correction of neglected clubfoot using the Ilizarov external fixator. Foot Ankle Int 2006;27:266–73.

50. Wallander H, Hansson G, Tjernström B. Correction of persistent clubfoot deformities with the Ilizarov external fixator. Experience in 10 previously operated feet followed for 2-5 years. Acta Orthop Scand 1996;673:283–7.

51. Franke J, Grill F, Hein G, et al. Correction of clubfoot relapse using Ilizarov's apparatus in children 8-15 years old. Arch Orthop Trauma Surg 1990;110:33–7.

52. Correll J, Forth A. Correction of severe clubfoot by the Ilizarov method. J Foot Ankle Surg 1996;2:27–32.

53. Oganesyan OV, Istomina IS, Kuzmin VI. Treatment of equinocavovarus deformity in adults with the use of a hinged distraction apparatus. J Bone Joint Surg Am 1996;784:546–56.

54. de la Huerta F. Correction of the neglected clubfoot by the Ilizarov method. Clin Orthop Relat Res 1994;301:89–93.

55. Oganesian OV, Istomina IS. Talipes equinocavovarus deformities corrected with the aid of a hinged-distraction apparatus. Clin Orthop Relat Res 1991;266:42–50.

56. Bradish CF, Noor S. The Ilizarov method in the management of relapsed club feet. J Bone Joint Surg Br 2000;82:387–91.

57. Grill F, Franke J. The Ilizarov distractor for the correction of relapsed or neglected clubfoot. J Bone Joint Surg Br 1987;69:593–7.
58. Grant AD, Atar D, Lehman WB. The Ilizarov technique in correction of complex foot deformities. Clin Orthop Relat Res 1992;280:94–103.
59. Kocaoğlu M, Eralp L, Atalar AC, et al. Correction of complex foot deformities using the Ilizarov external fixator. J Foot Ankle Surg 2002;41:30–9.
60. Eidelman M, Katzman A. Treatment of arthrogrypotic foot deformities with the Taylor Spatial Frame. J Pediatr Orthop 2011;31:429–34.
61. Eidelman M, Keren Y, Katzman A. Correction of residual clubfoot deformities in older children using the Taylor spatial butt frame and midfoot Gigli saw osteotomy. J Pediatr Orthop 2012;32:527–33.
62. Koczewski P, Shadi M, Napiontek M. Foot lengthening using the Ilizarov device: the transverse tarsal joint resection versus osteotomy. J Pediatr Orthop B 2002; 11:68–72.
63. Paley D. The correction of complex foot deformities using Ilizarov's distraction osteotomies. Clin Orthop Relat Res 1993;293:97–111.
64. Hosny GA. Correction of foot deformities by the Ilizarov method without corrective osteotomies or soft tissue release. J Pediatr Orthop B 2002;11:121–8.

The Indications and Technique for Surgical Correction of Pes Cavus with External Fixation

Kang Lee, MD[a], Jae-ho Cho, MD[b], Woo-Chun Lee, MD, PhD[b],*

KEYWORDS

- Pes cavus • Cavovarus • Foot deformity • Surgery • Osteotomy • External fixation
- Gradual correction

KEY POINTS

- Patients with severe and rigid cavovarus foot may suffer from pain and discomfort that may cause calluses, ulcerations, and fractures.
- The goal of treatment for severely deformed cavovarus foot is to provide a stable, painless, plantigrade foot.
- Treatment of severe cavovarus with progressive etiology, soft-tissue compromise, and coexisting deformities is challenging.
- Gradual correction with external fixation may be preferred as a first-line treatment option for severe and rigid cavovarus foot.

INTRODUCTION

Cavovarus is a deformity with abnormal elevation of the longitudinal arch, which consists of hindfoot varus and forefoot equinus. It is commonly associated with an underlying neuromuscular disorder, and an established diagnosis is crucial before planning treatment.[1] Cerebral palsy, spinal cord lesions with poliomyelitis, myelomeningocele, and peripheral neuropathies such as Charcot-Marie-Tooth (CMT) disease are common neuromuscular disorders that result in cavovarus deformity. These disorders induce cavovarus deformity as a result of long-standing muscle imbalance between the intrinsic and extrinsic muscles.[2] Intrinsic muscles of the sole become weak and later contracted, leading to abnormal elevation of the longitudinal arch.[3]

Funding Sources: None.

Conflict of Interest: None.

[a] Department of Orthopaedic Surgery, Kangwon National University Hospital, Kangwon National University, Baengnyeong-ro 156, Chuncheon 200-722, Republic of Korea; [b] Seoul Foot and Ankle Center, Inje University Seoul Paik Hospital, Mareunnae-ro 9, Jung-gu, Seoul 100-032, Republic of Korea

* Corresponding author.

E-mail address: wclee@seoulpaik.ac.kr

Residual clubfoot deformity is another cause of cavovarus deformity. The incidence of severe residual cavovarus deformity has decreased tremendously since the introduction of the Ponseti casting technique. However, neglected clubfeet are still being seen in developing countries, and recurrence of the deformity occurs frequently because of its complex pathoanatomy and clinical characteristics, even after appropriate treatment.[4,5]

Contracture after severe trauma may also cause cavovarus deformity.[6] Abnormality may result from ischemic contracture after compartment syndrome, from direct crushing injury to surrounding soft tissues, or as a consequence of neurovascular compromise.

Regardless of the cause, as the deformity become more severe and rigid, patients may suffer from pain and discomfort with decreased ambulatory capacity, instability, and gait abnormalities. If such conditions are untreated, calluses, soft-tissue ulcerations, fractures, and problems with the entire musculoskeletal system may develop.[2] Therefore, the goal of treatment should aim at converting a rigid and severely deformed cavovarus into a painless, stable, plantigrade foot.[7,8]

TREATMENT METHODS

Various methods can be used for the treatment of cavovarus foot, although no clear-cut guideline has been established. The method of treatment varies depending on the exact nature of the abnormality, and should be adopted to match each specific deformity. Conservative treatment does not have a significant role in the correction of such deformity. Surgical treatment consists of soft-tissue procedures, bony procedures, or a combination of both, stabilized with either internal or external fixation. In most patients, appropriate correction can be achieved with acute corrections using a combination of soft-tissue procedures and osteotomies. However, certain patients may require more radical procedures with high complication rates, such as primary triple arthrodesis, which may lead to reduced foot height and lower placement of malleoli.[7,9]

Gradual correction with external fixation has some advantages over acute correction in that it is less invasive and allows simultaneous correction of all components of the deformity separately.[10,11] Using osteotomies instead of bone resection, height loss of the foot can be reduced.[9] Direct assessment of soft-tissue viability during gradual correction is possible, and the amount and rate of correction can be modified accordingly.[7] Therefore, surgeons can expect predictably promising results without major complications.

INDICATIONS FOR EXTERNAL FIXATION

During the decision-making process for the treatment of cavovarus deformity, several factors may influence surgeons in deciding to make use of external fixation. First, cavovarus with underlying neuromuscular disorder that is often progressive form an ideal situation. According to Lee and colleagues,[7] young patients with lower motor neuron disease are at risk of substantial recurrence requiring additional surgical correction. Because of its progressive nature, incomplete elimination of neuromuscular imbalance may cause recurrence of the deformity. Hence, complete correction of all components or even overcorrection of the deformity is essential. However, precise acute correction of all the components of severely deformed cavovarus feet in young patients with progressive etiology is often very difficult even for an experienced specialist.[12]

Second, feet with cavovarus deformity caused by residual clubfoot or posttraumatic compartment syndrome tend to have severe joint stiffness and contraction of soft tissues. Extensive scar formation is common because many patients have undergone surgery at least once. There are potential risks for neurovascular injury, skin necrosis, infection, and ischemia after deformity correction.[13–16] Therefore, only a limited number of treatment methods are available for surgeons to choose from when treating rigid deformities with poor soft-tissue coverage.[17,18]

Third, existence of severe equinus deformity should be evaluated thoroughly. It has been reported that mild equinus deformities of approximately 10° may be corrected with acute lengthening procedures.[10] Although it may depend on the condition of surrounding soft tissues, the authors usually obtain full correction of equinus deformity of up to 20° with traditional heel-cord lengthening and posterior capsule release, with or without tibialis posterior lengthening. Additional procedures such as skin graft or flaps, tissue expanders, or shortening osteotomies should be considered in acute correction of larger equinus deformities.[1,19] Therefore it has been suggested to apply an external fixator when large corrections are necessary.[1,10]

Fourth, Complete physical examination of the entire lower extremity should be done to evaluate for any concomitant abnormality such as torsional malalignment or leg-length discrepancy. External tibial torsion is found at times in cavovarus deformity.[20] Overpowering the tibialis posterior muscle in CMT disease may act as external rotator of the tibia by inverting and internally rotating the foot. On the other hand, several patients with primary external tibial torsion may develop cavovarus deformity after habitual intentional internal rotation of the foot. Correction of cavovarus alone in these patients may lead to recurrence of the deformity, because they will intentionally rotate their foot to compensate for newly developed out-toeing gait. Such torsional malalignment may be corrected acutely with supramalleolar derotational osteotomy of the tibia. However, surgeons should always be cautious of nerve injury with acute derotations. The authors prefer gradual correction with external fixation if torsional malalignment exceeds 20° in adults.

Leg-length discrepancy may occasionally coexist with equinocavovarus deformity, and sometimes such a discrepancy may be the primary cause of equinus deformity. Therefore if leg-length discrepancy is not corrected simultaneously, equinus deformity may recur even after a perfect correction.

GRADUAL CORRECTION METHODS

Deformity correction with external fixation can be performed with either nonosteotomy or osteotomy techniques.[10,21] A nonosteotomy technique with gradual soft-tissue stretching is appropriate for young patients with only mild bony deformities,[8,16,22] although it has been reported that it is even possible to correct cavovarus deformities using an Ilizarov external fixator without any additional procedures in certain cases.[23] In general, a nonosteotomy technique is usually reserved for children younger than 8 years.[10,22,24] However, Grill and Franke[14] were able to treat 9 patients ranging in age from 8 to 15 years with severe equinocavovarus feet with an Ilizarov external fixator without any bone resection. Moreover, El-Mowafi and colleagues[17] achieved satisfactory results in teenagers treated for residual or recurrent clubfoot, with good bone morphology using nonosteotomy techniques.

In cavovarus foot with severe bony deformity, distraction of only soft tissues may often result in joint incongruity or recurrence of the deformity.[25,26] Such patients would benefit from osteotomy alone or in combination with other soft-tissue procedures.[10] The principle of deformity correction is to perform the osteotomy at the apex of the deformity. For instance, supramalleolar osteotomy is performed for deformities of the distal tibia.[27] Not only can it correct equinus/calcaneus and varus/valgus deformities, it is also very useful for correction of rotational malalignment and leg-length discrepancy. Variations of calcaneal osteotomy combined with osteotomy of talus and midfoot have been introduced for the treatment of severe cavovarus deformities (see later discussion).

The osteotomy technique may be further divided into osteotomy alone and osteotomy followed by secondary arthrodesis. Osteotomy without secondary arthrodesis may permit preservation of foot mobility, which eventually will allow better function. However, in severe deformities, especially with neuromuscular imbalance, secondary arthrodesis may be required to prevent recurrence.[7]

ALGORITHMIC APPROACH FOR CAVOVARUS CORRECTION WITH EXTERNAL FIXATION

Many surgeons consider gradual correction with external fixation to be the mainstay of treatment for patients with rigid severe cavovarus deformity. Nevertheless, there are only a few recently published studies in the English literature describing an algorithmic approach to the treatment of cavovarus deformity with external fixation. For neurologic equinocavovarus foot deformity, Lee and colleagues[7] recommended correcting the deformity step by step. First, hindfoot varus deformity should be evaluated. If the deformity is fixed, a Dwyer calcaneal osteotomy can be performed. Then the cavus component should be assessed. For moderate cavus deformity, plantar fasciotomy, abductor hallucis release, and first cuneiform plantar opening-wedge osteotomy is recommended. In addition, for severe pronation deformity, transcuneiform plantar opening-wedge osteotomy should be performed. For the remaining cavus, first metatarsal dorsal closing-wedge osteotomy may be additionally performed. Thereafter, cuboid lateral closing-wedge osteotomy can be added for any remaining forefoot adduction. However, midtarsal dorsal closing-wedge osteotomy along with plantar fascia and abductor hallucis release should be performed in very rigid and severe cavus deformity. The remaining deformities are then corrected gradually using external fixation.

Following this algorithm, Lee and colleagues[7] achieved satisfactory results in patients younger than 10 years. On the other hand, except in 1 case, adult patients with severe cavovarus deformity required secondary triple arthrodesis following this algorithm. The authors believe that osteotomy through one of the triple joints (eg, U-, V-, Y-osteotomy) from the beginning would be more appropriate for adults, rather than disrupting the midfoot and later performing a triple arthrodesis. Therefore, in the authors' opinion this algorithmic approach for neurologic cavovarus deformity should only be applied to children younger than 10 years (**Fig. 1**).

A recently study used a Taylor spatial frame (TSF) and midfoot osteotomy for correction of residual clubfoot deformities in teenagers.[28] These investigators achieved satisfactory results with initial midfoot osteotomy followed by TSF application and gradual correction. This study also evaluated hindfoot varus preoperatively, after which midfoot osteotomy was performed. The 3 calcaneal osteotomies performed at the time of frame removal should be considered as one of the additional procedures that are commonly performed for minor deformities that remain after extensive correction of deformity with external fixation.

Shalaby and Hefny[27] introduced an algorithm of decision making for the correction of complex foot deformities based on clinical and radiologic assessments. Various forms of osteotomies were performed in accordance with relationships between the leg, hindfoot, and forefoot.[27] This algorithm clinically defines equinus, heel varus or valgus, and cavus deformity. Then radiographic measurements are evaluated. With distal tibial abnormality, supramalleolar osteotomy should be performed. If there is

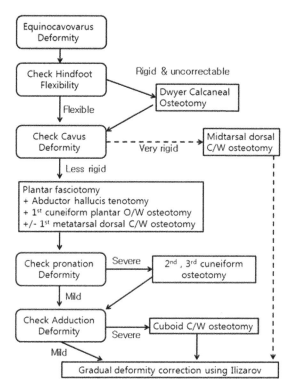

Fig. 1. Algorithmic flowchart for the treatment of neurologic equinocavovarus foot deformities using Ilizarov methods. C/W, closing wedge; O/W, opening wedge. (*From* Lee DY, Choi IH, Yoo WJ, et al. Application of the Ilizarov technique to the correction of neurologic equinocavovarus foot deformity. Clin Orthop Relat Res 2011;469:866; with permission.)

no ankle joint arthritis and the talar dome is normal, midtarsal osteotomy is performed when the relationship between forefoot and hindfoot is abnormal. In cases with ankle arthritis and flat-top talus, and an abnormal relationship between the leg and foot as a whole, U-osteotomy is indicated. However, if there are additional abnormal relationships between the forefoot and hindfoot, a V-osteotomy should be performed. Although the algorithm is relatively well described, this study shows only the result after a V-osteotomy. Therefore, one is unable to recognize or predict the results of midtarsal and U-osteotomy by following this algorithmic approach.

DISTRACTION OSTEOTOMIES

Using a Dwyer closing-wedge osteotomy, realignment of hindfoot varus can be achieved in only mild deformities.[29] Therefore, complex distraction osteotomy techniques such as U-osteotomy, V-osteotomy, and Y-osteotomy are required in severe cases. These techniques are usually indicated in very rigid and severely deformed cavovarus with stiff ankle joint and flat-top talus.[27]

U-Osteotomy

U-Osteotomy begins from the superior part of the calcaneus, passes underneath the subtalar joint, and crosses the sinus tarsi to the talar neck anteriorly. A plantigrade foot can be achieved with the ankle mortise undisturbed (**Fig. 2**). Foot height, equinus, calcaneus, varus, and valgus deformities can be corrected with U-osteotomy. However, because the U-osteotomy does not correct any deformity in the midfoot, it should be considered primarily when there is an abnormal relationship between the leg and the foot as a whole.[1,2,27]

V-Osteotomy

The V-osteotomy is a complex double osteotomy via the talus and calcaneus.[25] The osteotomy site may be exposed either through an Ollier approach or percutaneously.[24,27] Beginning from the midportion of plantar lateral surface of the calcaneus, the anterior cut runs anterodorsally across anterior and medial facets of calcaneus, exiting through the talar neck. The posterior cut lies posterior to the peroneal tendons, and is obliquely directed to exit on the calcaneus dorsal surface behind the posterior facet.[27] Both cuts should intersect with an angle of approximately 60° to 70° on the plantar surface of the calcaneus (**Fig. 3**).[21,30] It is crucial to always confirm that the osteotomies are complete, either by twisting an osteotome within the osteotomy space or by visualizing the cuts on the C-arm image intensifier.[21,27] V-Osteotomy is indicated when simultaneous correction of multiplanar deformities of hindfoot, midfoot, and forefoot are required.[21,27,30]

Y-Osteotomy

To perform Y-osteotomy, a curved submalleolar and small lateral incision is required.[30] An oblique posterior cut of the Y shape is made through the small lateral incision into the calcaneus. Then a vertical cut is performed, followed by an oblique anterior cut of calcaneus and talar neck. All 3 cuts should intersect with an angle of approximately 120°, mimicking a 3-ray star (**Fig. 4**). Y-Osteotomy has been reported to be exclusively corrective.[30] Because it has a larger cut surface with 3 planes of osteotomy, it requires a lesser degree of distraction, which may eventually lead to shorter healing time in comparison with V-osteotomy.

Unfortunately, it is very important to acknowledge that subtalar joint motion may become interrupted with the aforementioned distraction osteotomy techniques. Therefore, such a procedure should not be performed if there is normal subtalar motion unless secondary subtalar arthrodesis is planned. Meanwhile, by modifying the

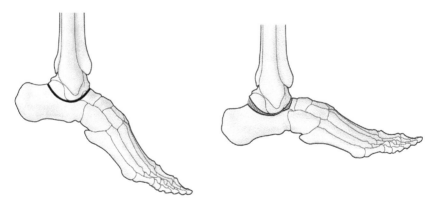

Fig. 2. Deformity correction with U-osteotomy. Osteotomy begins from the superior part of the calcaneus, passing underneath the subtalar joint, and crosses the sinus tarsi to the talar neck anteriorly.

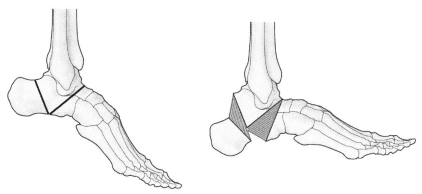

Fig. 3. Deformity correction with V-osteotomy. The anterior cut runs anterodorsally across anterior and medial facets of calcaneus, exiting through the talar neck. The posterior cut lies obliquely directed to exit on the calcaneus dorsal surface behind the posterior facet.[27] Both rims should intersect with an angle of approximately 60° to 70°.

anterior cut of V-osteotomy to cross through the cuboid-navicular or cuboid-cuneiform row, simultaneous midfoot osteotomy can be performed without disrupting the subtalar joint.[1]

EXTERNAL FIXATOR APPLICATION

Before application of the external fixator, it is very important to evaluate the vascularity of the foot, which can be done using angiography or Doppler ultrasonography. Neglected disruption of vascularity may later result in catastrophic amputation.[25] Moreover, if V-osteotomy or Y-osteotomy is planned, or when equinus correction should exceed 20°, the tarsal tunnel should be decompressed in advance to prevent dysesthesia following deformity correction.[1,2,25] Then soft-tissue procedures are performed followed by osteotomies such as Dwyer osteotomy and midtarsal osteotomy, with or without tendon transfer/tenotomy depending on each component of deformity.[7] In severe equinus contractures, lengthening of the Achilles may be performed as much as possible before application of the external fixator.

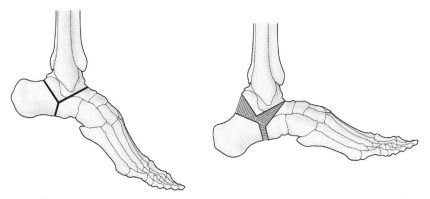

Fig. 4. Deformity correction with Y-osteotomy. All 3 cuts should intersect with an angle of approximately 120°, mimicking a 3-ray star.

The external fixator is divided into 2 assembly systems. The tibial assembly is constructed of a 2-ring block using transfixing wires (1.5 or 1.8 mm) and half pins (5 mm). The foot assembly is constructed with 1 or 2 half rings around the hindfoot a further 1 or 2 half rings for the forefoot.[8] Half rings around the hindfoot should be positioned parallel to the hindfoot sole in the coronal plane. Then threaded rods and hinges are assembled for correction of all components of deformity.

Under the concept that reduction of talonavicular joint and medial rotation of the talus will allow the deformed foot to approach normal, a transfixing olive wire is inserted into the talar neck from lateral to medial, perpendicular to the longitudinal axis of the talus.[8,31,32] By pulling the externally rotated talar head medially, the wire will allow derotation of the talus and thus restore the talocalcaneal angle (**Fig. 5**).[7,8] This process is similar to that during the Ponseti casting technique whereby the

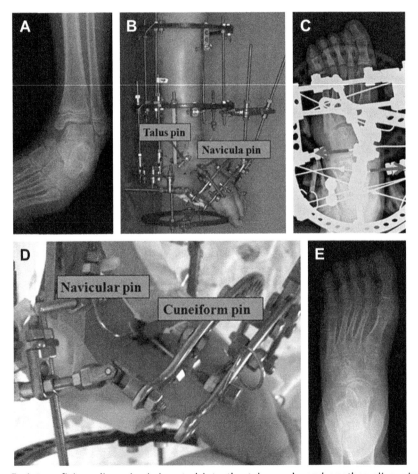

Fig. 5. A transfixing olive wire is inserted into the talar neck, and another olive wire is inserted into the navicular for reduction of talonavicular joint. After reduction of the talonavicular joint, the navicular olive wire is transposed to the tibial ring for distraction osteogenesis of midfoot osteotomy. (*From* Lee DY, Choi IH, Yoo WJ, et al. Application of the Ilizarov technique to the correction of neurologic equinocavovarus foot deformity. Clin Orthop Relat Res 2011;469:866; with permission.)

surgeon places the thumb on the talar neck. In addition, another olive wire can be inserted into the navicular from medial to lateral to facilitate talonavicular joint reduction.[7] After talonavicular joint reduction, transposition of navicular stirrup wire to the tibial ring is performed for distraction osteogenesis of the cuneiform osteotomy.[7] It is very important to be aware that reduction of the talonavicular joint through pulling the olive wire is only effective when subtalar and midtarsal joints are mobile. Therefore, in severe rigid bony deformities of the hindfoot or midfoot, additional bony procedures may be necessary.

Hindfoot equinus and varus can be corrected by distraction of rods connecting the tibial and hindfoot rings. To prevent the talus from impinging on the tibia, the hinge should be located posterosuperiorly from the ankle joint, and the ankle joint should be overdistracted during the process (**Fig. 6**). Forefoot adduction and midfoot cavus can be managed by distraction of rods between tibial and forefoot rings. During the correction, early weight bearing is very difficult with the severely deformed foot fixed to the bulky external fixator. Therefore, the patient may bear weight as tolerated with crutches once a plantigrade foot is achieved.

After achieving full correction of all deformities, the external fixator should be maintained for a few weeks in mild overcorrection, and the foot should be placed in a partial weight-bearing cast for another few weeks after removal of the fixator until the osteotomies have consolidated completely. If there is some remaining neuromuscular imbalance or joint incongruity, secondary arthrodesis should be performed.

COMPLICATIONS

The most common complication in surgery with external fixation is pin-site infection.[25,27,28,30] An association between wire tension, frame stability, and pin-site infections has been reported.[27] Skin tethering may also cause pin-site infections. Tented skin should be released with local anesthesia if severe pain or infection occurs.[33] On most occasions, oral antibiotics and careful monitoring of the pin site will be sufficient to treat pin-site infections. Occasionally, claw toes, which may occur after correction of severe deformity, can be prevented by foot support or insertion of transfixing pins. For children, separation of epiphysis can be a problem, which should be

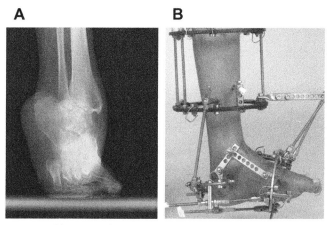

Fig. 6. (A) A 54-year-old man with severe equinocavovarus deformity caused by residual poliomyelitis. (B) The deformity was corrected with V-osteotomy and Ilizarov external fixation.

prevented with transfixing pins before distraction.[8,27] Other reported complications include premature consolidations, nonunions, dysesthesia, and vascular injuries, mostly caused by the rate and amount of distraction.

SUMMARY

Despite a significant increase in the range of motion, treatment of severe cavovarus foot with various techniques of external fixation improves patient satisfaction by achieving a painless plantigrade foot.[7–9,11,17,22,27,34]

Considering the varying etiology, possible neurovascular and other soft-tissue compromise, and coexisting deformities, treatment of a cavovarus foot is challenging, especially in severe cases. Often, acute correction may not be sufficient. In fact, severe vascular damage can occur with acute corrections, which may eventually lead to catastrophic amputation of the foot. Therefore, gradual correction with external fixation is preferred as one of the first-line-treatment options for such rigid and severe cavovarus deformities.

REFERENCES

1. Schrantz WF. Arthrogryposis. In: McCarthy JJ, Drennan JC, editors. The child's foot and ankle. 2nd edition. Philadelphia: Lippincott Williams and Wilkins; 2010. p. 250–7.
2. Kucukkaya M, Karakoyun O, Armagan R, et al. Correction of complex lower extremity deformities with the use of the Ilizarov-Taylor spatial frame. Acta Orthop Traumatol Turc 2009;43(1):1–6 [in Turkish].
3. Sabir M, Lyttle D. Pathogenesis of pes cavus in Charcot-Marie-Tooth disease. Clin Orthop Relat Res 1983;(175):173–8.
4. Dobbs MB, Rudzki JR, Purcell DB, et al. Factors predictive of outcome after use of the Ponseti method for the treatment of idiopathic clubfeet. J Bone Joint Surg Am 2004;86(1):22–7.
5. Haft GF, Walker CG, Crawford HA. Early clubfoot recurrence after use of the Ponseti method in a New Zealand population. J Bone Joint Surg Am 2007;89(3): 487–93.
6. Perry MD, Manoli A 2nd. Reconstruction of the foot after leg or foot compartment syndrome. Foot Ankle Clin 2006;11(1):191–201, x.
7. Lee DY, Choi IH, Yoo WJ, et al. Application of the Ilizarov technique to the correction of neurologic equinocavovarus foot deformity. Clin Orthop Relat Res 2011; 469(3):860–7.
8. Choi IH, Yang MS, Chung CY, et al. The treatment of recurrent arthrogrypotic club foot in children by the Ilizarov method. A preliminary report. J Bone Joint Surg Br 2001;83(5):731–7.
9. Kucukkaya M, Kabukcuoglu Y, Kuzgun U. Management of the neuromuscular foot deformities with the Ilizarov method. Foot Ankle Int 2002;23(2):135–41.
10. Paley D. The correction of complex foot deformities using Ilizarov's distraction osteotomies. Clin Orthop Relat Res 1993;(293):97–111.
11. Paley D, Lamm BM. Correction of the cavus foot using external fixation. Foot Ankle Clin 2004;9(3):611–24, x.
12. Schwend RM, Drennan JC. Cavus foot deformity in children. J Am Acad Orthop Surg 2003;11(3):201–11.
13. McKay DW. New concept of and approach to clubfoot treatment: section III— evaluation and results. J Pediatr Orthop 1983;3(2):141–8.

14. Grill F, Franke J. The Ilizarov distractor for the correction of relapsed or neglected clubfoot. J Bone Joint Surg Br 1987;69(4):593–7.
15. Ferreira RC, Costo MT, Frizzo GG, et al. Correction of neglected clubfoot using the Ilizarov external fixator. Foot Ankle Int 2006;27(4):266–73.
16. Grant AD, Atar D, Lehman WB. The Ilizarov technique in correction of complex foot deformities. Clin Orthop Relat Res 1992;(280):94–103.
17. El-Mowafi H, El-Alfy B, Refai M. Functional outcome of salvage of residual and recurrent deformities of clubfoot with Ilizarov technique. Foot Ankle Surg 2009; 15(1):3–6.
18. Steinwender G, Saraph V, Zwick EB, et al. Complex foot deformities associated with soft-tissue scarring in children. J Foot Ankle Surg 2001;40(1):42–9.
19. Ohmori S. Correction of burn deformities using free flap transfer. J Trauma 1982; 22(2):104–11.
20. Hansen ST. The cavovarus/supinated foot deformity and external tibial torsion: the role of the posterior tibial tendon. Foot Ankle Clin 2008;13(2):325–8, viii.
21. Samchukov ML, Cherkashin AM, Rodriguez E, et al. Stepwise approach to equinus deformity correction with circular external fixation. In: Cooper PS, Polyzois VD, Zgonis T, editors. External fixators of the foot and ankle. Philadelphia: Lippincott Williams and Wilkins; 2013. p. 391–408.
22. Kocaoglu M, Eralp L, Atalar AC, et al. Correction of complex foot deformities using the Ilizarov external fixator. J Foot Ankle Surg 2002;41(1):30–9.
23. Hosny GA. Correction of foot deformities by the Ilizarov method without corrective osteotomies or soft tissue release. J Pediatr Orthop B 2002;11(2):121–8.
24. El-Mowafi H. Assessment of percutaneous V osteotomy of the calcaneus with Ilizarov application for correction of complex foot deformities. Acta Orthop Belg 2004;70(6):586–90.
25. Segev E, Ezra E, Yaniv M, et al. V osteotomy and Ilizarov technique for residual idiopathic or neurogenic clubfeet. J Orthop Surg (Hong Kong) 2008;16(2):215–9.
26. Bradish CF, Noor S. The Ilizarov method in the management of relapsed club feet. J Bone Joint Surg Br 2000;82(3):387–91.
27. Shalaby H, Hefny H. Correction of complex foot deformities using the V-osteotomy and the Ilizarov technique. Strategies Trauma Limb Reconstr 2007;2(1): 21–30.
28. Eidelman M, Keren Y, Katzman A. Correction of residual clubfoot deformities in older children using the Taylor spatial butt frame and midfoot Gigli saw osteotomy. J Pediatr Orthop 2012;32(5):527–33.
29. Dwyer FC. The present status of the problem of pes cavus. Clin Orthop Relat Res 1975;(106):254–75.
30. Kirienko A, Peccati A, Abdellatif I, et al. Correction of poliomyelitis foot deformities with Ilizarov method. Strategies Trauma Limb Reconstr 2011;6(3):107–20.
31. Carroll NC. Controversies in the surgical management of clubfoot. Instr Course Lect 1996;45:331–7.
32. Carroll NC, McMurtry R, Leete SF. The pathoanatomy of congenital clubfoot. Orthop Clin North Am 1978;9(1):225–32.
33. Slomka R. Complications of ring fixators in the foot and ankle. Clin Orthop Relat Res 2001;(391):115–22.
34. Ferreira RC, Costa MT, Frizzo GG, et al. Correction of severe recurrent clubfoot using a simplified setting of the Ilizarov device. Foot Ankle Int 2007;28(5): 557–68.

Arthrodesis for the Cavus Foot
When, Where, and How?

Jacob R. Zide, MD, Mark S. Myerson, MD*

KEYWORDS

- Arthrodesis • Cavus • Cavovarus deformity • Foot

KEY POINTS

- A well-done arthrodesis that creates a plantigrade foot is superior to a joint-sparing surgery that preserves limited motion but fails to gain complete correction.
- Midfoot arthrodesis is ideally suited for the anterior cavus foot in which the apex of the deformity is located distal to the transverse tarsal joint.
- Soft tissue balancing is a vital part of deformity correction, a well performed triple arthrodesis will tend to recur without appropriate tendon transfers.
- The best outcomes involve minimal shortening of the foot, therefore correction should be by rotation and translation with minimal wedge resection.

INTRODUCTION

Management of the cavus foot is challenging and as the foot assumes a rigid posture, surgical options become more limited. Depending on the location of the deformity's apex, midfoot or triple arthrodesis tend to be the mainstays of treatment once the foot has lost its flexibility. In general, these are viewed as salvage operations and are used for the foot that is too far gone for correction by joint-sparing means. Arthrodesis should not be thought of as a salvage procedure; it is rare for an arthrodesis to significantly impair functional ability in this patient group even if there is a flexible deformity. Although maintaining motion is one of the goals of reconstruction, the results of a well-done arthrodesis that creates a plantigrade foot are superior to those of a joint-sparing surgery that preserves a limited amount of motion but fails to gain complete correction.

The literature is replete with reports, cases, and studies of failure of arthrodesis, but this is the result of incomplete correction or correction that was not associated with corrected muscle balance. It is not sufficient to rely on bony correction (in this instance, arthrodesis) alone. Soft tissue balancing, by means of tendon transfers, must be included in the correction. A comprehensive understanding of the muscular forces, remaining flexibility of the foot, location of the apex (or apices) of deformity,

The authors have nothing to disclose.
The Institute for Foot and Ankle Reconstruction, Mercy Medical Center, 301 St. Paul Place, Baltimore, MD 21202, USA
* Corresponding author.
E-mail address: mark4feet@aol.com

Foot Ankle Clin N Am 18 (2013) 755–767
http://dx.doi.org/10.1016/j.fcl.2013.08.012

and available surgical procedures to effect the solution are paramount to achieving reliable outcomes.

CLINICAL EVALUATION

A complete neurologic examination with special attention paid to the assessment of muscle strength is essential in the clinical evaluation of the cavus foot. The problem is dynamic (and often progressive), so it planning for tendon balancing is a necessary part of the correction. Although this is well known in the setting of the joint-sparing procedures for flexible cavus, it has often been overlooked when treating the rigid deformity. It has been our observation that, without proper soft tissue balancing, bony procedures alone are likely to fail.

In the classic cavovarus deformity the major deforming forces are the tibialis posterior and the peroneus longus, which overpower the peroneus brevis and tibialis anterior, respectively.[1] This imbalance leads to the varus hindfoot and pronated and plantarflexed medial column commonly encountered. However, this muscle imbalance is never the same for different patients, and the final changes in muscle power that may or may not be present a decade following the reconstruction cannot be predicted. Therefore, variations in muscle strength are always encountered and evaluation of their relative differences is critical. The prototypical tendon transfer for the cavus foot is to use the posterior tibial tendon and place it in a position that is beneficial for the foot and ankle, particularly with respect to regaining some dorsiflexion power. However, muscle power of any commonly transferred tendon in the cavus foot, particularly the posterior tibial, is variable. When the muscle is weak, surgeons are typically loath to use it as a tendon transfer, judging it too weak or insufficient for transfer. However, this thought process creates a setup for failure because there is always some power left in the muscle that will overcome its antagonist and gradually lead to recurrence of deformity.

The next consideration is to evaluate the rigidity of the deformity. The classic clinical test of rigidity is the Coleman block test. In this test, the lateral forefoot and heel rest on a block of wood, while the plantarflexed first ray is lowered off the edge of the block. If hindfoot varus remains uncorrected after removing the plantarflexed first ray from the equation, then the hindfoot varus is said to be rigid.[2] The challenge to effectively and predictably using this test is that there is a spectrum to flexibility and rigidity, and it is difficult to know what to do when the hindfoot partially corrects. Although the Coleman block test can establish whether there is some flexibility, it does not allow the examiner to judge how correctable the hindfoot is.

The Coleman block is not the only way to assess hindfoot rigidity and others have suggested maneuvers for evaluating hindfoot flexibility while the patient is non–weight bearing. One method is performed by placing the patient in a prone position with the knee flexed at 90°. In this position, the foot is allowed to move freely without the influence of the first ray, and hindfoot manipulation is easily performed, allowing determination of rigidity.[3] Although a test of rigidity while weight bearing is relevant, it is not as useful as the impression that clinicians obtain when examining the foot in the seated position. We therefore always perform the examination of the foot by manipulating the heel with the patient in a seated position and the foot dangling from the examination table. This method allows the examiner to better evaluate the amount of retained hindfoot motion, and it is easier to perform than the Coleman block test or by having the patient lie prone.[4] With this method, if the heel is correctable to a valgus position then, regardless of what happens to the forefoot, there is still the possibility that an arthrodesis can be avoided. If the hindfoot is only partially correctible it is our practice to choose arthrodesis rather than trying a joint-sparing procedure because a well-aligned fusion yields superior outcomes to an osteotomy that leaves the foot undercorrected.

Standard anteroposterior, oblique, and lateral weight-bearing radiographs of the foot and ankle are obtained to evaluate the cavus foot deformity. Perhaps the most important of these images is the weight-bearing radiograph of the ankle. We take it for granted that the foot will be deformed, but the ankle ultimately determines the outcome of the result of correction. Angular radiographic evaluation includes evaluation of the calcaneal pitch, Meary angle, and Hobbs angle, which are helpful in quantifying the amount of deformity.[5] Determining the apex of the deformity, which is nearly always multiplanar, is the most important guiding factor in deciding where the correction needs to be focused. The location of the apex in the sagittal plane is used to determine whether the deformity is an anterior (midfoot) or posterior (hindfoot) cavus, but correction in the coronal plane must also be planned for. Understanding the three-dimensional nature of the cavus deformity allows clinicians to plan for correction of equinus, abduction or adduction, and rotational malalignment (**Fig. 1**).

The hindfoot alignment view is a useful adjunct in radiographic evaluation. It is helpful in measuring the amount of deformity present and can provide an objective gauge of the amount of correction of hindfoot varus achieved after surgical intervention (**Fig. 2**). We do not routinely obtain advanced imaging but a computed tomography scan could be considered to evaluate arthritic change of the involved joints and to further define the deformity.

DEFORMITY CORRECTION

The sagittal apex is either the midfoot or the hindfoot, and determines the location as well as the type of the procedure. Whatever is done to correct one plane of deformity has an impact on the other planes as well. The medial column of the foot is always

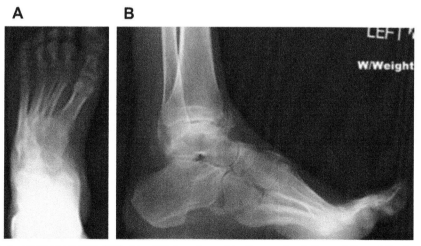

Fig. 1. Anteroposterior (AP) view (*A*) showing adduction and rotation of the midfoot and forefoot with obvious subluxation of the talonavicular joint resulting from imbalance of the stronger tibialis posterior against the weaker peroneus brevis. Lateral view (*B*) showing cavovarus deformity with the fibula externally rotated and posterior while the subtalar joint is internally rotated. The rotation of the midfoot gives the appearance that the navicular sits on top of the cuboid. There is equinus of the medial column as a result of the peroneus longus overpowering the tibialis anterior.

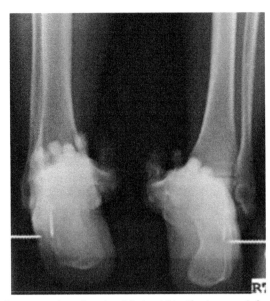

Fig. 2. Hindfoot alignment view showing bilateral hindfoot varus deformity.

more plantarflexed than the lateral column, but the lateral column tends to be more fixed, rotated, and adducted. Thus, when correcting the plantarflexion of the first ray, rotational malalignment must also be addressed or the foot will be left with continued overload of the lateral column.

It is our practice to perform posterior tibial tendon transfer to the cuboid or lateral cuneiform and peroneus longus to brevis transfer as a matter of routine, regardless of the type of arthrodesis chosen. If not transferred, the midfoot arthrodesis fails because overpull by the tibialis posterior causes adductus at the level of the talonavicular joint. With a triple arthrodesis, the broad insertion of the posterior tibial tendon leads to progression of heel varus. In either setting, a new apex of deformity is created by the intact insertion of the tendon (**Fig. 3**).

The peroneus longus to brevis transfer is also a vital part of the overall procedure. Without release of the longus, recurrence of first metatarsal plantarflexion occurs whether midfoot or triple arthrodesis is performed. We routinely transfer the peroneus longus to the weakened peroneus brevis for added eversion and dorsiflexion power. In addition, the insertion of the anterior tibial tendon may need to be transferred laterally. Even though it is being overpowered by the peroneus longus, the tibialis anterior often still has strength and contributes to the deformity by creating a dorsal midfoot apex. Without release and transfer of the tendon it may be impossible to unwind the foot adequately for correction.

Midfoot Arthrodesis

Midfoot arthrodesis is ideally suited for the anterior cavus foot in which the apex of the deformity is located distal to the transverse tarsal joint. Triple arthrodesis is unable to correct the forefoot equinus present in this deformity and is therefore the incorrect procedure in this situation.

Concerns about wound healing, nonunion, and technical difficulty of the operation have led surgeons to avoid midfoot arthrodesis. However, failure to use this powerful procedure creates a situation in which the surgeon attempts to control the deformity

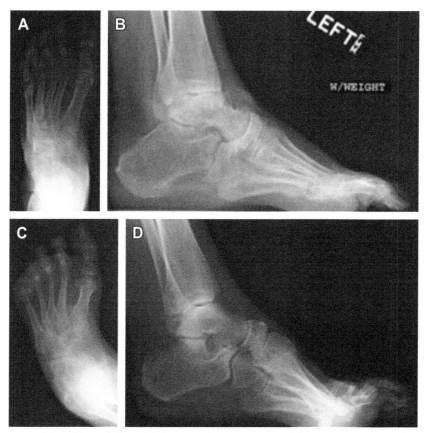

Fig. 3. AP (*A*) and lateral views (*B*) showing classic cavovarus deformity with the tibialis posterior as the main deforming force. AP (*C*) and lateral views (*D*) showing midfoot cavus with the peroneus longus overpowering the tibialis anterior creating the main deforming force.

from a point distant from its apex, which makes it difficult (if not impossible) to achieve satisfactory correction. We disagree with this method of management and have found that, with careful handling of the soft tissues and meticulous surgical technique, these are rare complications.

Several techniques have been described, including the Akron midtarsal dome osteotomy[6] and several dorsal wedge osteotomies. Jahss[7] described performing a dorsal wedge at the level of the tarsometatarsal joints, whereas Cole[8] and Japas[9] performed a dorsal wedge osteotomy at the naviculocuneiform/cuboid level.

Our preferred technique has been that put forth by Japas,[7] because this does not shorten the foot, it provides correction at the apex of the deformity, and it allows for multiplanar correction; that is, plantarflexion and adductus (**Fig. 4**). The midfoot arthrodesis must be performed with a release of the plantar fascia.

An extensile dorsal midline incision from the ankle to the midmetatarsal is created. The superficial peroneal nerve is retracted laterally and the deep peroneal nerve and dorsalis pedis artery are elevated via a subperiosteal plane and taken medially. Tenotomy of the extensor hallucis brevis tendon may be necessary in order to gain access to the midfoot. The entirety of the dorsal central midfoot is then stripped with a periosteal

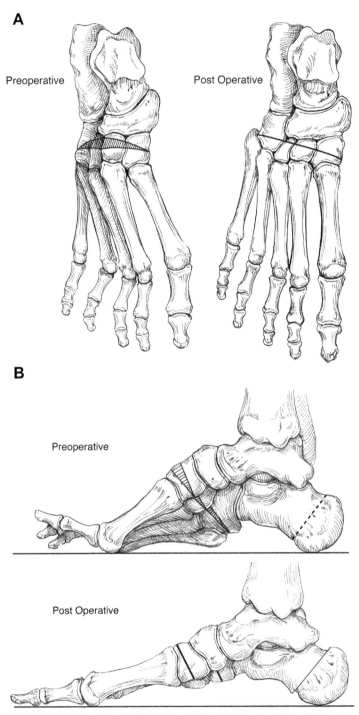

Fig. 4. (A) The authors' preferred technique for midfoot arthrodesis. The medial and lateral wedges shown on the AP view allow correction of the plantarflexion of the medial column and the rotation and adduction of the lateral column. (B) The lateral view shows the dorsally based wedges taken from the midfoot. A calcaneal osteotomy is often included in the procedure to help with correction of the calcaneal pitch and heel varus.

elevator. The sagittal apex of the deformity is identified fluoroscopically and a saw is used to perform the osteotomy. The osteotomy usually exits its medial limb in the medial cuneiform so the anterior tibial tendon needs to be reflected out of the way. The lateral limb generally exits in the cuboid but this depends on the amount of rotational and angular correction required. The limbs of the osteotomy meet at an apical point, typically the middle cuneiform. More of a dorsal wedge needs to be removed medially than laterally; the medial correction is achieved mostly by dorsiflexion through the wedge resection, whereas the lateral correction is done by dorsal translation and rotation. If adductus needs to be corrected in addition to the cavus, biplanar correction is achieved by resecting slightly more bone dorsally and laterally. The forefoot is corrected through a combination of dorsiflexion, elevation, and rotation. If necessary, the medial column can be reduced first, mostly through dorsiflexion, and held in place with a temporary k-wire. This technique allows correction of the lateral column through translation and rotation, which can be stabilized with a second temporary k-wire. Once good bony apposition has been achieved, the type of fixation can be determined. Screws, plates, or percutaneous Steinmann pins may be used for fixation, and the decision of which to use is made during the surgery and is based on the amount of bone remaining for purchase of the hardware as well as the overall quality of the bone. We do not recommend staples, because there is often inadequate bone for fixation on either side of the osteotomy. Once the osteotomy has been stabilized, the tendon transfer(s) can be completed. We typically plug the posterior tibial tendon into the cuboid or the lateral cuneiform and perform a peroneus longus to brevis tenodesis. If plate fixation is selected, the tendon transfer(s) can be completed by passing the tendon under the plate and securing the sutures to the plate or sewing the tendon back on itself. Otherwise, the posterior tibial tendon can be inserted through a bone tunnel and held with a tenodesis screw or held with a suture anchor.

Triple Arthrodesis

For the rigid posterior cavus deformity, triple arthrodesis has historically been the procedure of choice, but this procedure on its own may not be sufficient to correct a multiplanar deformity or one with multiple apices of deformity (**Fig. 5**). This surgery is a daunting procedure for the inexperienced surgeon and thorough surgical planning and consideration of a staged procedure is necessary.

As mentioned previously, it has been our observation that a triple arthrodesis performed without soft tissue rebalancing often recurs. Published results of the triple arthrodesis for cavus foot deformity show variable outcomes. Santavirta and colleagues[10] reviewed 15 consecutive patients (26 feet) treated for Charcot-Marie-Tooth

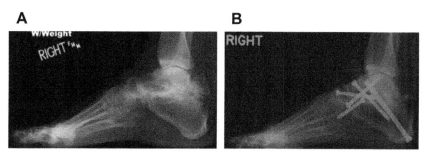

Fig. 5. Cavus deformity with hindfoot apex and severe hindfoot arthritis (A) treated with triple arthrodesis (B).

with various foot and ankle fusions. Twenty-one of the feet were treated with triple arthrodesis at an average age of 21.7 years (range, 11–61 years). Six of these feet underwent concomitant soft tissue procedures and 5 feet in 3 patients needed subsequent soft tissue procedures to improve foot balance after healing. They reported 15 good to excellent results and 6 fair to poor results in the patients having triple arthrodesis and noted that the patients who were followed for greater than 15 years did not have a substantially higher number of poor results than those followed for less time.

Wukich and Bowen[11] followed 34 feet (22 patients) that underwent triple arthrodesis for pes cavovarus for an average of 12 years, 7 months. The average patient age in their study was 16 years, 10 months. Thirty-one of the 34 feet (19 of 22 patients) were satisfied with the results of their surgery, but they also reported that 22 of the feet also had continued pain and 19 feet had plantar callosities. The investigators further noted that residual deformity, including cavus, varus, and cavovarus, was present in 15 of 34 feet (45%). Three of the patients in their series required a drop foot brace after surgery. None of these three patients had undergone a posterior tibial tendon transfer at the time of the index surgery and, as a result, the investigators began routinely including this procedure.[11] The author point is that they relied on the fusion without balancing the muscular forces. Even with a well-performed triple, there are still forces on the midfoot, such as the tibialis posterior, tibialis anterior, and peroneus longus imbalance, and the long extensors, which continue to act as deforming forces if left in place (**Fig. 6**).

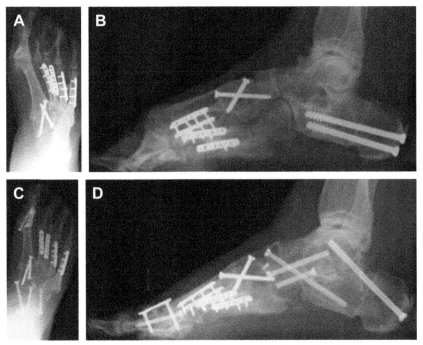

Fig. 6. AP (*A*) and lateral views (*B*) showing a patient who had undergone a previous attempt at reconstruction without appropriately addressing the deforming force of the tibialis anterior leading to the dorsal bunion deformity. The patient required revision (*C, D*) with triple arthrodesis and transfer of the anterior tibial tendon to the midfoot.

Wetmore and Drennan[12] reported the longest follow-up. They followed 30 feet in 16 patients for an average of 21 years (range, 6–51 years). This study reported 20% fair and 46% poor results; outcomes that were significantly worse than others reported in the literature. Persistent varus and cavus were noted in 9 feet, and recurrence of cavovarus occurred in 7 feet (23%) that had originally been correctly aligned. The number of patients with a poor outcome increased with the length of time after their procedure. They recommended that triple should be reserved as a salvage procedure and necessitates the adjunctive use of muscle-balancing procedures to reduce the risk of recurrence.[12] The results of this study should serve as a warning to the surgeon who plans to rely on bony correction alone for the cavus foot. They show what is bound to happen without the addition of soft tissue procedures. We strongly believe that these types of outcomes can be avoided when the appropriate balance of the foot is achieved at the time of surgical correction.

These studies show the challenges inherent in obtaining and maintaining correction without soft tissue balancing. Cavovarus deformities tend to be both dynamic and progressive and only a well-balanced foot is stable over time. Soft tissue balancing contributes to the long-term success of the arthrodesis, because it removes the major deforming forces going forward.

There are several techniques of triple arthrodesis described in the literature. The original description by Hoke[13] used a lateral incision and fused only the subtalar and talonavicular joints. He described making a cut through the neck of the talus and removing the head and neck in preparation for arthrodesis. The neck portion had to be shortened because, when the equinus deformity was corrected with dorsiflexion, the head and neck piece was too long to go back in.[13] Ryerson's[14] technique involves taking a wedge from the transverse tarsal joint for correction of transverse or sagittal plane deformity. Lambrinudi's[15] technique creates a notch in the posteroinferior portion of the navicular and then an oblique cut through the talar head. The cut surface of the neck of the talus is then plantarflexed down to the anterior process of the calcaneus and wedged under the notch that was made in the navicular. The angle produced posteriorly by the flexed talus on the calcaneus is filled with the bone graft piece obtained from the talar head and neck.[15]

The beak triple arthrodesis was described by Siffert and colleagues[16] specifically for correction of the cavus deformity. In this technique, the dorsal cortex of the navicular is removed. An osteotomy of the anterior calcaneus and talar head and neck are performed in order to create the talar beak. The forefoot is then displaced downward and the navicular is locked under the talar beak for correction of the deformity.[16] Despite its appearance, this arthrodesis gains length of the foot. It works extremely well when the apex is dorsal, directly at the talonavicular joint.

Our method of triple arthrodesis for the cavus foot is to use medial and lateral incisions, keeping in mind the exposure that will be required for later tendon transfers. The lateral incision is begun at the tip of the fibula and extended distally toward the base of the fourth metatarsal long enough to expose the calcaneocuboid (CC) joint. It is important to watch for the sural nerve during the dissection and it should be retracted plantarward along with the peroneal tendons. The extensor digitorum brevis is retracted dorsally and the soft tissues are elevated sharply from the floor of the sinus tarsi. The sinus tarsi is then distracted with a toothed laminar spreader allowing visualization of the interosseous ligament, which can be sharply divided and removed with a rongeur, allowing access to the posterior and middle facets of the subtalar (ST) joint. Preparation of the ST joint is with a 1-cm flexible chisel used to denude the cartilage, and then a curved osteotome is used to rigorously fish-scale the surfaces of the middle and posterior facets. Next, a large periosteal elevator is used to strip the lateral surfaces of the calcaneus and cuboid at the level of the CC joint. The peroneal retinaculum is retracted inferiorly and a knife is swept vertically through the CC joint and rotated dorsally through the bifurcate ligament. Plantarflexion and supination of the forefoot by an assistant often affords excellent visualization of the CC joint but a small laminar spreader can also be used if necessary. Preparation of the joint is performed in the same manner as for the ST joint. We achieve the corrected position of the ST and CC joints through rotation and translation, but it is extremely rare that removal of a bone wedge is necessary and we try to avoid this whenever possible. The talonavicular (TN) joint is exposed via a medial incision extending from the ankle to the medial cuneiform lying just medial to the anterior tibial tendon. The extensor retinaculum is incised and the anterior tibial tendon is retracted laterally. The posterior tibial tendon is prepared for transfer at this time by release of its insertion. It is important to preserve as much length of the tendon for transfer as possible by following and releasing its insertion onto the medial cuneiform and first metatarsal distally. Subperiosteal dissection around the TN joint is performed medially and dorsally. A laminar spreader is used to distract the joint for preparation. Because the medial column is already short in the cavus foot deformity, it is vital that a minimum of bone resection be performed while still gaining excellent preparation for arthrodesis. After the cartilage is denuded with a chisel, we often use a burr in order to break through the subchondral plate while still maintaining the overall shape of the joint.

The TN joint is most often the apex of the hindfoot cavus deformity. For this reason, the TN joint is reduced first by rotation, abduction, and dorsiflexion. Provisional pinning of the TN joint is performed and the position of the heel is then assessed and corrected at the subtalar joint to approximately 5° of valgus (in some severe cases, the heel varus is so significant that a lateralizing calcaneal osteotomy has to be added to the procedure in order to gain enough correction for adequate positioning of the heel). This correction is also held with provisional guide pin fixation. The TN joint is then fixed with 2 5.5-mm cannulated, partially threaded screws or a single screw and dorsal 2-hole locking compression plate depending on the quality of the bone and the purchase and compression achieved by the first screw. The medial compression screw is inserted first from distal to proximal, beginning at the medial tuberosity of the navicular. It is important to make sure that the screw head is flush with the margin of the joint so it does not protrude into the naviculocuneiform joint. In most instances we then place a dorsal 2-hole locking compression plate over the central aspect of the TN joint. Sometimes the lateral TN joint gaps open slightly after placement of the medial compression screw, making it preferable to use a second screw instead of a plate. If a second screw is chosen, then it is placed percutaneously from the dorsolateral aspect of the navicular. Fixation of the subtalar joint is then performed with a partially threaded 7.0-mm screw inserted from the heel (but off the weight-bearing surface of the calcaneus) into the body of the talus. Fixation of the CC joint is then performed. The cuboid has a tendency to subluxate plantarward and, if fixed in this position, it tends to cause lateral column pain with weight bearing. It is therefore vital to elevate the lateral forefoot to make sure that the plantar surface of the cuboid is even with that of the calcaneus on the lateral fluoroscopic view before fixation. The CC joint can be fixed from in an antegrade or retrograde fashion. A 5.5-mm screw is placed across the joint, usually from proximal to distal, after creating a lateral notch in the calcaneus approximately 1 cm proximal to the CC joint in order to recess the screw head. If screw purchase or compression across the joint is poor, a 4-hole locking plate can be applied to the dorsolateral surface of the joint for added stability and compression. Sometimes, even though the CC joint has been reduced completely, the rotation of the forefoot is such that the base of the fifth metatarsal is still very plantar. In

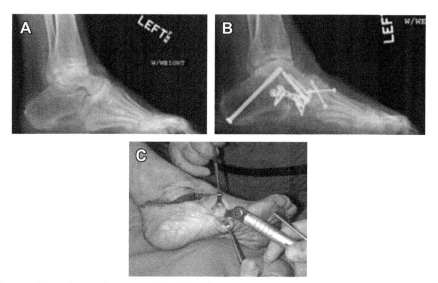

Fig. 7. This patient, who required triple arthrodesis and arthrodesis of the first tarsometa-tarsal joint, also had a painful callus overlying the base of the fifth metatarsal. The preop-erative lateral view (*A*) shows the rotated position of the fifth metatarsal with the base lying significantly inferior to the cuboid. Postoperative lateral view (*B*) after excision of the base of the fifth metatarsal. The excision (*C*).

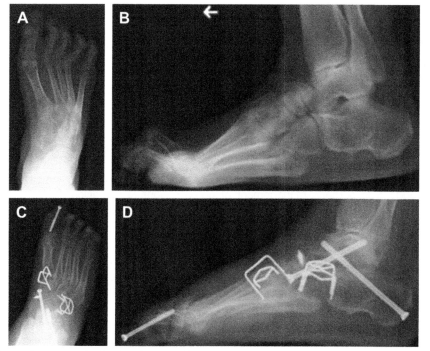

Fig. 8. This patient had a double apex of deformity with cavovarus stemming from both the hindfoot and the midfoot (*A, B*). The patient was treated with both midfoot and triple arthrodesis as well as transfer of the anterior tibial tendon and extensor hallucis longus (*C, D*).

this case, ostectomy of the plantar surface or complete excision of the base of the fifth metatarsal should be performed to relieve lateral column overload. The peroneus brevis has a broad insertion and it is generally unnecessary to release the tendon from the base of the metatarsal. However, if the tendon is released in its entirety, it can be sewn along with the peroneus longus into the periosteum of the lateral aspect of the cuboid (**Fig. 7**).

At this point, stability of the ankle should be assessed, because it may be necessary to add a Chrisman-Snook procedure to correct lateral ligament instability. Transfer of the posterior tibial tendon to the cuboid or lateral cuneiform is then completed, as is the peroneus longus to brevis transfer (**Fig. 8**).

SUMMARY

When the cavus foot has become rigid, midfoot and triple arthrodesis may be the only reasonable surgical options left. The apex of the deformity is multiplanar and some deformities may have more than one apex. The best outcomes are achieved with minimal shortening of the foot, so correction should be by rotation and translation and with minimal wedge resection wherever possible.

In the past, persistent deformity and recurrence have been a major problem after correction of the rigid foot because of a lack of understanding of the importance of soft tissue balance. It is not enough to focus on the hindfoot even if this is where most of the deformity is present, and leaving the midfoot or forefoot alone is certain to result in recurrence. Posterior tibial tendon transfer and peroneus longus transfer are nearly always required for correction, and other soft tissue procedures (such as anterior tibial tendon transfer, plantar fascia release, tendo-achilles lengthening, and gastrocnemius slide) may be necessary as well. If the principles of soft tissue balancing are followed, arthrodesis is an excellent procedure despite the literature that states to the contrary.

REFERENCES

1. McCluskey WP, Lovell WW, Cummings RJ. The cavovarus foot deformity. Etiology and management. Clin Orthop Relat Res 1989;(247):27–37.
2. Coleman SS, Chesnut WJ. A simple test for hindfoot flexibility in the cavovarus foot. Clin Orthop Relat Res 1997;(123):60–2.
3. Price BD, Price CT. A simple demonstration of hindfoot flexibility in the cavovarus foot. J Pediatr Orthop 1997;17(1):18–9.
4. Myerson MS. Cavus foot correction. In: Myerson MS, editor. Reconstructive foot and ankle surgery: management of complications. 2nd edition. Philadelphia: Elsevier; 2010. p. 155–73.
5. Aminian A, Sangeorzan BJ. The anatomy of cavus foot deformity. Foot Ankle Clin 2008;13:191–8.
6. Wilcox PG, Weiner DS. The Akron midtarsal dome osteotomy in the treatment of rigid pes cavus: a preliminary review. J Pediatr Orthop 1985;5(3):333–8.
7. Jahss MH. Tarsometatarsal truncated-wedge arthrodesis for pes cavus and equinovarus deformity of the fore part of the foot. J Bone Joint Surg Am 1980;62(5):713–22.
8. Cole WH. The treatment of claw-foot. J Bone Joint Surg Am 1940;22(4):895–908.
9. Japas LM. Surgical treatment of pes cavus by tarsal V-osteotomy. Preliminary report. J Bone Joint Surg Am 1968;50(5):927–44.
10. Santavirta S, Turunen V, Ylinen P, et al. Foot and ankle fusions in Charcot-Marie-Tooth disease. Arch Orthop Trauma Surg 1993;112(4):175–9.

11. Wukich DK, Bowen JR. A long-term study of triple arthrodesis for correction of pes cavovarus in Charcot-Marie-Tooth disease. J Pediatr Orthop 1989;9(4): 433–7.

12. Wetmore RS, Drennan JC. Long-term results of triple arthrodesis in Charcot-Marie-Tooth disease. J Bone Joint Surg Am 1989;71(3):417–22.

13. Hoke M. An operation for stabilizing paralytic feet. J Orthop Surg 1921;3: 494–507.

14. Ryerson EW. Arthrodesing operations on the feet. J Bone Joint Surg Am 1923;5: 453–71.

15. Lambrinudi C. New operation on drop-foot. Br J Surg 1927;15:193–200.

16. Siffert RS, Forster RI, Nachamie B. "Beak" triple arthrodesis for correction of severe cavus deformity. Clin Orthop Relat Res 1966;45:101–6.

Index

Note: Page numbers of article titles are in **boldface** type.

Foot Ankle Clin N Am 18 (2013) 769–792
http://dx.doi.org/10.1016/S1083-7515(13)00094-6
1083-7515/13/$ – see front matter © 2013 Elsevier Inc. All rights reserved.

foot.theclinics.com

United States Postal Service
Statement of Ownership, Management, and Circulation
(All Periodicals Publications Except Requestor Publications)

1. Publication Title	2. Publication Number	3. Filing Date
Foot and Ankle Clinics of North America	0 1 6 - 3 6 8	9/14/13

4. Issue Frequency	5. Number of Issues Published Annually	6. Annual Subscription Price
Mar, Jun, Sep, Dec	4	$299.00

7. Complete Mailing Address of Known Office of Publication (Not printer) (Street, city, county, state, and ZIP+4®)

Elsevier Inc.
360 Park Avenue South
New York, NY 10010-1710

Contact Person
Stephen R. Bushing

Telephone (Include area code)
215-239-3688

8. Complete Mailing Address of Headquarters or General Business Office of Publisher (Not printer)

Elsevier Inc., 360 Park Avenue South, New York, NY 10010-1710

9. Full Names and Complete Mailing Addresses of Publisher, Editor, and Managing Editor (Do not leave blank)

Publisher (Name and complete mailing address)

Linda Belfus, Elsevier, Inc., 1600 John F. Kennedy Blvd. Suite 1800, Philadelphia, PA 19103-2899

Editor (Name and complete mailing address)

Jennifer Flynn-Briggs, Elsevier, Inc., 1600 John F. Kennedy Blvd. Suite 1800, Philadelphia, PA 19103-2899

Managing Editor (Name and complete mailing address)

Adrianne Brigido, Elsevier, Inc., 1600 John F. Kennedy Blvd. Suite 1800, Philadelphia, PA 19103-2899

10. Owner (Do not leave blank. If the publication is owned by a corporation, give the name and address of the corporation immediately followed by the names and addresses of all stockholders owning or holding 1 percent or more of the total amount of stock. If not owned by a corporation, give the names and addresses of the individual owners. If owned by a partnership or other unincorporated firm, give its name and address as well as those of each individual owner. If the publication is published by a nonprofit organization, give its name and address.)

Full Name	Complete Mailing Address
Wholly owned subsidiary of	1600 John F. Kennedy Blvd, Ste. 1800
Reed/Elsevier, US holdings	Philadelphia, PA 19103-2899

11. Known Bondholders, Mortgagees, and Other Security Holders Owning or Holding 1 Percent or More of Total Amount of Bonds, Mortgages, or Other Securities. If none, check box ☒ None

Full Name	Complete Mailing Address
N/A	

12. Tax Status (For completion by nonprofit organizations authorized to mail at nonprofit rates) (Check one)
The purpose, function, and nonprofit status of this organization and the exempt status for federal income tax purposes:
☐ Has Not Changed During Preceding 12 Months
☐ Has Changed During Preceding 12 Months (Publisher must submit explanation of change with this statement)

PS Form 3526, September 2007 (Page 1 of 3 (Instructions Page 3)) PSN 7530-01-000-9931 PRIVACY NOTICE: See our Privacy policy in www.usps.com

---

13. Publication Title	14. Issue Date for Circulation Data Below
Foot and Ankle Clinics	September 2013

15. Extent and Nature of Circulation			Average No. Copies Each Issue During Preceding 12 Months	No. Copies of Single Issue Published Nearest to Filing Date
a. Total Number of Copies (Net press run)			839	902
b. Paid Circulation (By Mail and Outside the Mail)	(1)	Mailed Outside-County Paid Subscriptions Stated on PS Form 3541. (Include paid distribution above nominal rate, advertiser's proof copies, and exchange copies)	542	617
	(2)	Mailed In-County Paid Subscriptions Stated on PS Form 3541 (Include paid distribution above nominal rate, advertiser's proof copies, and exchange copies)		
	(3)	Paid Distribution Outside the Mails Including Sales Through Dealers and Carriers, Street Vendors, Counter Sales, and Other Paid Distribution Outside USPS®	124	136
	(4)	Paid Distribution by Other Classes Mailed Through the USPS (e.g. First-Class Mail®)		
c. Total Paid Distribution (Sum of 15b (1), (2), (3), and (4))		▶	666	753
d. Free or Nominal Rate Distribution (By Mail and Outside the Mail)	(1)	Free or Nominal Rate Outside-County Copies Included on PS Form 3541	43	60
	(2)	Free or Nominal Rate In-County Copies Included on PS Form 3541		
	(3)	Free or Nominal Rate Copies Mailed at Other Classes Through the USPS (e.g. First-Class Mail)		
	(4)	Free or Nominal Rate Distribution Outside the Mail (Carriers or other means)		
e. Total Free or Nominal Rate Distribution (Sum of 15d (1), (2), (3) and (4))		▶	43	60
f. Total Distribution (Sum of 15c and 15e)		▶	709	813
g. Copies not Distributed (See instructions to publishers #4 (page #3))		▶	130	89
h. Total (Sum of 15f and g)		▶	839	902
i. Percent Paid (15c divided by 15f times 100)			93.94%	92.62%

16. Publication of Statement of Ownership
☐ If the publication is a general publication, publication of this statement is required. Will be printed in the December 2013 issue of this publication.   ☐ Publication not required

17. Signature and Title of Editor, Publisher, Business Manager, or Owner

Stephen R. Bushing – Inventory Distribution Coordinator

Date   September 14, 2013

I certify that all information furnished on this form is true and complete. I understand that anyone who furnishes false or misleading information on this form or who omits material or information requested on the form may be subject to criminal sanctions (including fines and imprisonment) and/or civil sanctions (including civil penalties).

PS Form 3526, September 2007 (Page 2 of 3)

Moving?

Make sure your subscription moves with you!

To notify us of your new address, find your **Clinics Account Number** (located on your mailing label above your name), and contact customer service at:

Email: journalscustomerservice-usa@elsevier.com

800-654-2452 (subscribers in the U.S. & Canada)
314-447-8871 (subscribers outside of the U.S. & Canada)

Fax number: 314-447-8029

Elsevier Health Sciences Division
Subscription Customer Service
3251 Riverport Lane
Maryland Heights, MO 63043

Printed and bound by CPI Group (UK) Ltd, Croydon, CR0 4YY

03/10/2024

01040478-0018